ISBN: 978-1-7342924-0-4

Library of Congress Control Number: 2019918741

Wolf Vollmer Publishing
1813 Penn Ave,
Reading, PA, 19609

www.DrDeanWolf.com

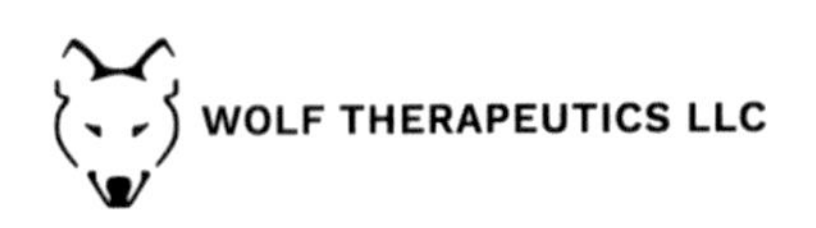

Get Lean with Dr. Dean

A doctors guide to...

Eating Healthier

Training Smarter

Preventing & Treating Injury

By: Dr. Dean Wolf

Contents

Preface..........7

Chapter 1
Diet..........10

Chapter 2
Supplements..........35

Chapter 3
Orthotics..........52

Chapter 4
The Cause of Joint Pain..........63

Chapter 5
Weight training..........85

Chapter 6
Aerobic Exercise..........112

Chapter 7
Tendonosis..........125

Chapter 8
Spinal injury, prevention and treatment..........131

Chapter 9
Extremity injury, prevention and treatment..........168

Chapter 10
Health care and alternative treatments..........219

Preface

The reason I decided to write this book was that, after 30 years of practice and hundreds of thousands of patient encounters, I found it surprising how many people didn't know how to go about getting back into shape. I've trained every kind of athlete imaginable and given nutritional advice to many professional athletes, including NFL and MLB players. I remember a week in which I saw two different physicians as patients who each asked questions that surprised me. One was doing some form of circuit training and after 2 months wasn't getting any stronger. He was working out Monday, Wednesday, and Friday, doing the same exercises every day without much result. The other doctor came to me with a knee issue and told me he was using heat and taking an anti-inflammatory medication. I said to myself, "If these two doctors, who are well-trained, do not understand basic fundamental principles of working out and rehabilitation, then how many other people could benefit from this information?"

In this book I am going to tell you the secret to dieting correctly. I'll explain the differences between foods that help your diet and foods that don't. I will discuss what role vitamins and supplements play. I am going to teach you to identify predispositions for injury and how to fix them, or train around them. I am going to teach you how to work out with weight training and aerobic exercise. The simple do's and don'ts that will get you ripped in your 40s, 50s and beyond.

Not only will I discuss the injuries you might already have, I'll also focus on how to prevent other injuries from occurring. You will recognize the importance of alternative treatment regimens such as chiropractic care, nutritional supplementation, and the use of therapeutic supports. Moreover, you will be able to determine if you can treat your individual injuries with the knowledge from this book versus seeking professional medical care.

Through the years, one of the things that has driven me crazy about reading books is how many of them are full of extraneous or redundant material. The sum of most books could be four or five pages of material. I am the Mayor of Realville. Everything in this book is authentic and works because I've tried it and I've taught others who have also seen results. This self-help book is written in a unique way. The first part of each chapter will have the fundamental action plan. If that plan is sufficient, you can skip to the next chapter. The second part of each chapter will be called "Nuts and Bolts" and will have additional detailed explanations on what we discussed, as well as some reference tables, etc. For example, Section 5 of the Nuts and Bolts of Chapter 1 deals with medications that can slow down or otherwise affect weight loss. If you don't take medications for any conditions, why waste time reading this part? If we are in the injury sections of Chapter 8 and 9 and you don't have that specific problem, skip ahead to read something that is unique to your needs. You will have the flexibility to maneuver through the book efficiently. It is designed to be read in a few hours, or 15 hours if need be, all depending on how much extra relevant information you'd like. You may find that some chapters pertain to you now, while other chapters will be crucial down the road through the years.

A large part of taking care of ourselves and recovering from setbacks is having the right tools for the job. From both my personal and professional experience, I will explain the "hows and whys" of health products that really work, such as braces, supports, and supplements. I will also provide links to purchase these products at affordable prices.

Lastly, I am not going to try to impress you with my intellect. Instead, I am going to give you the real goods. You WILL NOT read sentences like this: "After engaging in several weeks of frequent increases of metabolic activity with progressive durations of physiologic cardiac stress and mechanical muscle loading, one will experience an increase in endorphins and enkephalins and will notice an overall enhancement of one's cosmetic appeal." On the other hand, you will read sentences like this: "After a few weeks of working out you will notice that you feel great and look great." Now, let's get into shape!

CHAPTER ONE

Diet

It's the Calories

Everyone likes to try different diets, searching for the magical answer to losing weight. Here's the bottom line: if you eat more calories than you burn, you gain weight. If you burn more calories than you eat, you lose weight. It's as simple as that. A calorie is the amount of energy that it takes to raise the temperature of 1 gram of water 1° Celsius. Nothing more, nothing less. It's just an energy measurement. 1 lb of body fat is equal to 3,500 calories. When you're trying to lose or maintain an ideal weight, I recommend keeping a count of your calories as opposed to tracking the number of grams of carbohydrates or fat. It's simpler and you don't need to have a Ph.D. in biochemistry.

I've exercised my entire life. Still, in my early 40s, I had weighed as much as 265 lbs. One of the most undeniable truths of life is that you cannot "out-exercise" a bad diet. I was very active, but simply eating more calories than my body was burning. Bodybuilders have said for years that diet is 75% of bodybuilding.

After seeing the following picture, I had enough of being out of shape. So, in 8 months I lost 80 lbs. Here's how I did it.

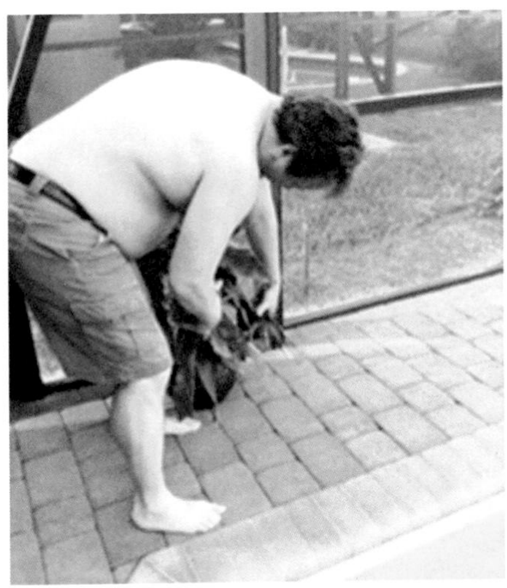
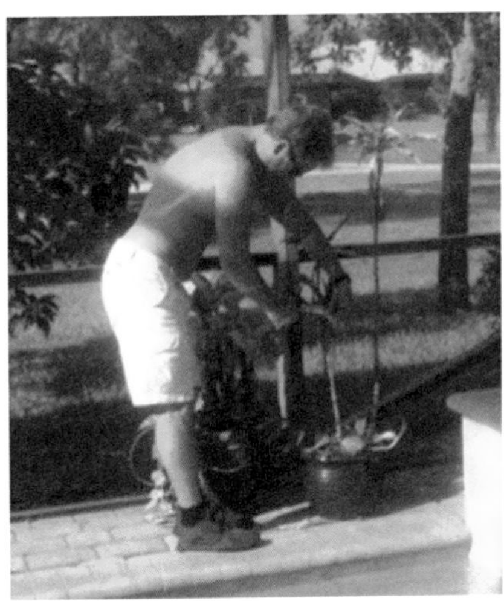

For me, one of the most useful tools was a fitness app on my phone. For 1 month, every single thing that I ate and drank, I logged into my app. I admit that it was cumbersome; however, it was a good way to get a grasp on how much I was eating. For instance, I knew foods like chicken wings are high in calories, but I didn't appreciate just how many calories. After a long day at work, it wasn't uncommon for me to go out for a dozen wings and a few beers with some friends. Unfortunately, in one partial meal, you take in 1,200 calories for the wings and another 200 calories for two light beers. If I went to the gym, got on the elliptical trainer, and was moving along at a pretty good pace, it would take me 2 solid hours to work off a dozen wings and two beers. Looking back, I couldn't believe how many calories I was unknowingly consuming. It didn't seem excessive, but when I looked at the numbers it was rare that I consumed any less than 3,000 calories in a day. No wonder I was overweight.

The challenge to dieting is to find a diet that you're most comfortable with. One of the more popular diets right now is the ketogenic diet. Even on a ketogenic diet, if you eat more calories than you burn, you will gain weight. I tried the keto diet. I liked the results. However, I found it difficult to stay with that diet. I like my carbs. On a personal level, I found one of the drawbacks to being in ketosis was a decreased aerobic performance at the gym. The nice thing about the keto diet is when your body gets into ketosis, it burns fat as a primary fuel source. An amazing side effect is that when your body is burning fat, you have less hunger. Hence, the popularity of that diet. I think the difference with this diet versus others is that it does reduce hunger. Therefore, reducing your calorie intake for the day. Once again, the most important thing is to have less caloric intake then caloric output, so choose whichever plan works best for you.

Another popular dieting choice is the 40/40/20 diet, meaning that 40% of your diet is going to be carbs, 40% protein intake, and 20% fat. I don't care for this one, for the same reason I don't like using an abacus or calculator to figure out the percentages and ratios of fat, carbs, and protein that I eat every meal.

I'm not a big fan of vegetarian or vegan diets. Some of the most unhealthy patients I have treated are vegetarians. I know this is going to get some people's feathers ruffled; I'm just telling it how it is. We need protein to build muscle. Most people who choose this lifestyle do not get enough protein. There is no doubt that you can get protein via vegetable sources, but it is much more difficult. You are not going to build mass on a vegan diet.

In fact, I believe the biggest flaw of almost all diets is the fact that the person is not getting enough protein. Have you ever noticed that people who lose a lot of weight look very frail and weak? Those people have lost a lot of muscle mass. That's what happens with most diets.

I could bore you by critiquing every diet out there. We need to try to figure out a way to lose weight and maintain the ideal body weight that you want. At the same time, you'll need a functional plan to stay at this weight for the rest of your life. So, here are seven gold standard tips for weight loss and weight stabilization.

Seven Tips For Losing Weight

1. Make sure you are healthy enough to lose weight with exercise.

First and foremost, get a physical. Make sure that you are able to start doing some physical exercise. Additionally, a good workup by a doctor could exclude physical disorders that handicap your ability to get back in shape. This physical should include a blood pressure test and an EKG. I recommend getting routine blood work that would include a CBC, a biochemical profile showing your blood sugars, a thyroid panel, and a complete lipid profile. (1) Once it's been determined you are good to go, we can start with the following tips.

2. Portion Control.

Chances are the most popular diets you see on TV include portion control – the ones that have you subscribing to their meal plans. I think these diets are expensive. However, it's a good way to understand how portion control can play a role in reducing your calories. This is not rocket science. If you lack self-discipline, these diets are not a bad way to go. Since we have established that the secret to losing weight is not to eat more calories than you burn, it's reasonable to be conscious of the fact that even eating clean low calorie foods can make you gain weight if you eat a large quantity. Therefore, it's important to have a degree of portion control, make sure you know how many calories a particular food has per serving to avoid eating too many calories.

3. Make Strategic Food Substitutions.

There are certain foods that are so high in calories that indulging in them makes losing weight so much more difficult. I consider the highest calorie troublemakers to be bread, pasta, and any form of a potato. These foods are problems metabolically for many biochemical reasons. However, for the purpose of this book, in my experience if your goal is to lose weight, you need to stay away from these three forms of food. If you're maintaining weight, you can have these on occasion. A nice healthy 6-inch sub at Subway has 320 calories in the whole wheat bread alone. A cup of pasta is 220 calories and we haven't even mentioned what we're going to put on the pasta. There are more carbohydrates in a baked potato than there are in a Snickers bar. These carbohydrates break down into sugar in your body and raise your blood glucose levels quickly. I find breakfast to be easy to prepare without using the high-calorie trouble makers. Any form of eggs or dairy products is a great way to start your day. My favorite go-to item is nutrient-rich plain Greek yogurt. It's low in carbs, high in protein, and low in calories. Lean meats should be the staple of the lunch and dinner menu. They have a huge amount of low-calorie, muscle-building protein. They are a much better choice than high-fat red meats. And when it comes to carbs you can't go wrong with complex carbohydrates over the simple carbohydrates that are found in bread and pasta. Main sources include fruits and most vegetables. Some examples are broccoli, cauliflower, beans, peas, and lentils. There is a more complete list in Section 6 of the Nuts and Bolts portion of this chapter.

4. Watch the food toppings!

Condiments on certain foods can make a huge difference in the amount of calories you eat during a week. For example, I found that I like mustard just as much as I like mayonnaise on a turkey sandwich. It's 550 calories with 2 tablespoons of mayonnaise and only 350 calories with 2 tablespoons of mustard. If you made one food substitution like this every day you would save 1,400 calories a week. Salad dressings are hidden landmines of dieting. The choice of salad dressings is important. Generally, the creamier it is, the more calories. After a short time, you will start noticing how much higher the calories are just by the texture of some of the things you're eating. Most salad dressings like; Thousand Island, French, Italian, and honey mustard are between 60 and 80 calories per tablespoon. And how many of us really use only 1 tablespoon? The vinaigrettes tend to be a little bit lower at around

40 calories per tablespoon. I try to find a low-calorie or low-fat dressing that is usually around 10 calories per tablespoon. So, if you put just 2 tablespoons of honey mustard dressing on your salad, you were adding 150 calories versus 2 tablespoons of light Italian at 20 calories. That's another 130 calorie difference for the day and another 810 calories for the week. I just had a nice salad today at my favorite restaurant and ordered balsamic vinaigrette on the side. They put it in this nice little black plastic cup. I took a tablespoon and scooped 7 tablespoons of dressing out of that cup! Holy cow! I would have lost that bet every day of the week and twice on Sunday. If that was Thousand Island dressing, it could have been another 400 calories! That's more calories than a half a pound of chicken breast! There's no better way to blow up a diet than with the wrong salad dressing choices.

The next huge offender is ketchup. It is 25% sugar. Ketchup is roughly 15 calories per tablespoon. Who uses 1 tablespoon of ketchup on anything? I would easily use 3-5 tablespoons of ketchup on a hot dog or a hamburger. On french fries, I'd start with 3 or 4 tablespoons. When I'm halfway finished with the fries, I'll add a couple more tablespoons. I put a chart of the most common condiments, dressings, and sauces in the Nuts and Bolts section of this chapter. It's good to look at them to get a feel for what foods are the major offenders. (2)

5. *Drinks.*

What are you drinking? I've found that when I'm trying to drop pounds, the only thing I drink is water, though sometimes I will drink some skim milk with a scoop of whey protein before I work out. Of course many of us like our caffeine. Brewed coffee only has 2 calories, but you have to watch what you put in it. We have a list of the coffee condiments in the Nuts and Bolts section of this chapter. (3) If you're drinking soda, you're drinking weight gain in a can. As a rule of thumb, a can of soda is 150 calories. I had a patient in my office that was drinking four sodas a day and was 100 lbs overweight. Just simply dropping the four cans of soda a day would account for 4,200 fewer calories a week, which equates to about 63 lbs weight loss in a year. I have to admit I like cola. I remember the first time I drank diet cola, I didn't care for the taste. It is amazing how you can get used to something different after a period of time. Now, I love diet cola. Sometimes, I'll have a diet cola in the afternoon to get my caffeine fix. Remember, it's the calories. A lot of ice tea products and other flavored drinks are loaded with sugar and high in calories. So, it's important to read your labels. As for alcohol, that is a difficult one. If you're trying to drop weight, you're going to have to limit your alcohol consumption. Personally, I won't drink any alcohol when I'm trying to lose weight. As a rule of thumb, spirits – Vodka, Rum, Tequila, Gin and Whiskey – average about 70 calories per ounce. Watch out for vodka and cranberry drinks or gin and tonics. Those mixers add another 100 calories or more to the spirit. A single rum and diet cola could be as little as 70 calories. Your best bang for the buck for mixers with alcohol is diet soda or club soda. They are both great alternatives when you want to drink alcohol and are trying to lose weight. Light beers average around 100 calories with some of the ultra low carb beers being as low as 85 calories. Regular beers average between 130 and 150 calories and higher. Typically, the higher the alcohol, the higher the calories. Red and white wines average around 120 calories per 5 ounce glass. Of course, the sweet dessert wines can be 200 calories per 5 ounce glass.

6. Weigh yourself every day.

Most diet plans suggest to weigh yourself once a week. I think it's better to weigh yourself every day. I like to get immediate feedback relative to what I ate and how I exercised the day before. If I'm not getting the desired weight loss, I might up my cardio or decrease my caloric intake. Of course, it's important to weigh yourself at the same time every day; preferably, first thing in the morning. Get a good digital scale. You get what you pay for. Be very consistent with your fluid intake at night time. I recommend not drinking anything 8 hours before your morning weigh in. The key is to get up in the morning and do your bathroom duties at about the same time every day and then weigh yourself so you can accurately track your gains or losses.

When I kick start a weight loss regimen, usually, my plan is to lose 30 lbs in 3 months. I like to get it over with. If you are eating correctly, you should be losing .2 to .3 lbs a day. Personally, I have found that to be a good pace. I admit that it is aggressive but not enough to slow down your metabolic rate. (4) When I'm targeting weight loss, I try to lose 10 lbs a month. Everyone will have to adjust their own weight loss to their comfort level. Not to mention, we all have different physiologies. Diabetes, thyroid disorders or other illnesses can affect your ability to lose weight. Certain medications can also impede weight loss. (5) Orthopedic injuries can limit your ability to exercise, thereby reducing an important avenue when trying to lose weight.

7. Get a Fitness Tracker.

Get a fitness tracker or some kind of smart watch. The beauty of these tools is that they are amazingly accurate. You can monitor your activity, sleep, and heart rate. If you haven't tried one of these, you don't know what you're missing. By entering your age, sex, height, and weight, these devices figure out how many calories you are burning each day. You can use this to determine how many calories you can eat. If you want to lose .3 lbs a day, you're going to have to burn 1,000 more calories than you eat. It sounds difficult but once you start tracking things, you'll find you can do it easily. A person with an active lifestyle could be burning 3,500 calories a day. With that kind of output, you would be able to eat 2,500 calories a day to lose .2-.3 lbs a day.

It's good to know what your metabolic rate is so we can determine how many calories you can eat. You could do this by finding your basal metabolic rate, which is the amount of calories you burn at rest, this is the energy used to simply keep your body functioning. The textbooks say that the average woman in the United States has a basal metabolic rate of 1,400 calories a day, while a man's is 1,800 calories a day. You can calculate your rate using the "textbook" method as follows: Women 655 + (4.35 x weight in lbs) + (4.7 x height in inches) - (4.7 x age in years). Men 66 + (6.23 x weight in lbs) + (12.7 x height in inches) - (6.8 x age in years). You would then take your basal metabolic rate and add it to the calories you spent during physical activity to get your total metabolic rate. Like the 40/40/20 diet, this seems sort of complex, doesn't it? This is way too complicated.

This is what I recommend doing. Get a fitness watch and make sure you have enter all of the important information, including your age, height, weight, and sex. Weigh yourself. Do this for 7 days to get solid numbers. If your weight doesn't change in 1 week, your fitness watch will tell you how many calories a day you burned on average. That is your metabolic rate. This way is much easier than doing complex math equations. In addition, your metabolic rate is dynamic. It will start to change for the better as you become more active. Everyone is different, and in situations like this, our metabolisms are going to change as we get more active. Once you know your base rate, you will know the caloric adjustments you will have to make to lose weight. Another natural way of boosting your metabolism is through the use of a few herbs. For metabolism increases, I like Ashwagandha (**wolfashwag.com**), Garcinia (**wolfgarcinia.com**), and Green Tea Extracts. (**wolfoxyburn.com**)

Know What Foods are What

Everything you consume can be divided into one of four categories: water, carbohydrates, fats, or proteins. Simply put, water is for physiological cellular transport. Water is used in all cells, organs, and tissues to help regulate chemistry, temperature, and maintain other bodily functions. Carbohydrates and fats are what your body uses for fuel. Protein is used to build tissue – everything, including the skin, muscle tissue, and organs. Let's discuss each one of these individually.

A) Carbohydrates

Carbohydrates are your primary fuel source. Simply put, carbohydrates are sugars. Simple sugars such as sucrose, which is basically table sugar, are metabolized into fuel very quickly. Another simple carbohydrate is fructose, which is the kind of sugar found in fruits. Fructose digests slower than sucrose because of the presence of fiber in fruits. Complex carbohydrates are sugars that are even more difficult for the body to break down into fuel. Complex carbohydrates are found in vegetables, grains, and legumes. This is my favorite sugar. Because of their complexity, it takes longer for the body to digest them and turn it into sugar. The longer it takes to turn into sugar, the slower the insulin response.

Let's talk about how the pancreas regulates blood sugar. Normally, I would put this in the Nuts and Bolts section of this chapter; however, I think it's important to understand the fundamental principles of glucose and insulin regulation in the body.

Here's how it works. When you eat food, the digestion processes turn the food into sugar. We don't need to make this overly technical by trying to determine the chemical differences between glucose, glycogen, and so on. So, let's just call it "sugar" for now. Sugar is the fuel source that our bodies use to make energy. Sugar is also caustic to a lot of tissues of the body. Therefore, high sugar levels in the bloodstream create damage to the body. Our bodies have to keep sugar levels in check to avoid disease. The pancreas creates insulin to maintain a safe blood sugar level. Quite simply, insulin lowers blood sugar. One bad thing about insulin is that it impedes body fat from being used as fuel. When we eat something very sugary, the pancreas must make insulin to lower the spike in blood sugar levels. Not to mention that when insulin is present, body fat will be stored rather than used for energy. When eating a french fry, your body breaks the potato down quickly, causing an insulin spike that sends all of the french fry's fat to your belly for storage for a rainy day. The quicker the spike in sugar levels, the more acute the pancreatic response of insulin. I will talk later in Chapter 5 about how to use this insulin response to our advantage when building muscle. We want to avoid the yo-yo effect of high sugar and consequent high insulin. All of us at one time or another have eaten a bunch of junk food and then felt awful a half hour later. That's because insulin levels rose and consequently another drop in blood sugar occurred. Usually, if you feel tired or sleepy after lunch, that's a sign that you ate too many carbs. The key here is to eat as many slow-burning carbohydrates as possible. They are more filling and lower in calories, giving you more energy and endurance. I list a table of great healthy carbs to put in your diet in the Nuts and Bolts section. (6) I have found a blend of different herbs, vitamins, and minerals that can help support normal blood sugar levels(**wolfstablesugar.com**). Ashwagandha (**wolfashwag.com**) and Garcinia (**wolfgarcinia.com**) herbal compounds have also been known to help aid blood sugar stabilization.

Here's an example of three different food choices with three different energy and consequential weight gain results. We will start with my all-time favorite cookie, the Girl Scouts Caramel deLites. Have you ever eaten five of them? Not hard to do. Well, five of those cookies equate to roughly 50 grams of carbohydrates and 350 calories. We won't even talk about the 20 grams of fat. Two small to medium apples have 50 grams of carbohydrates but only 180 calories; half the amount of the cookies. Let's say you ate four apples to equal the calories of the five cookies – do you think you'd want more apples? Of course not. That's because your insulin is not screaming to your brain that you are not satisfied. Green beans are a complex carbohydrate. You would have to eat 700 grams or 10 ½ cups of green beans to equal 50 grams of carbohydrates. If you could have eaten that many green beans, you would have taken in only 315 calories. See the difference in how our bodies react to these three foods? The crazy thing here is that after eating five cookies I could eat more. My insulin would be spiking right away, lowering my blood sugar, and my brain would be getting messages saying to eat more because my sugar is getting low. This is the yo-yo effect that is responsible for a mega-calorie diet and resultant weight gain.

B) Fats

Fats are an excellent fuel source. A gram of fat is 9 calories of energy and a gram of both carbohydrates and protein are 4 calories. Generally speaking, your unsaturated fats are better than saturated fats. Hydrogenated fats are clearly the worst for us and something we should avoid altogether, the reason being that hydrogenated fats contain trans fats. These are unhealthy fats because they raise our bad cholesterol and lower our good cholesterol.

I think fats stereotypically get a bad rap. The omega-3 fatty acids have long been linked to improved heart & vascular health. (wolfomega3.com) Most monounsaturated and polyunsaturated fats can be very healthy to eat. Look at the people in the Mediterranean area who have fat as a high source of their caloric intake. Their mortality rates are no different than ours in the United States. Olive oils and nuts are a great source of monounsaturated fats with many positive health benefits. Polyunsaturated fats found in vegetable oils and flaxseed oils, just to name a couple, have additional health benefits. One thing to watch with these types of oils is to avoid high-temperature frying. Studies have shown that there are harmful by-products with this kind of cooking. I avoid any kind of fried foods when I'm trying to get ripped. As a rule of thumb, fried foods are about 10% higher in calories as the same food grilled.

The Atkins diet and ketogenic diets that are popular right now can be a very healthy way of achieving weight loss. These diets highlight fat as the primary source of fuel for your diet. Personally speaking, I like to get my healthy fats from cheese, eggs, nuts, seeds, olive oils, and lean meats. For the purposes of weight loss, I like to trim as much fat out of my diet as possible. (7)

C) Protein

Protein is where the rubber meets the road in my book. Bodybuilders have known for years that if you want to get big, you have to eat. The more you eat, the bigger you get. My main focus when I'm trying to get ripped is protein consumption. For me, it's easier to keep track of. Additionally, it focuses on better eating habits. The gold standard I go by is 1 gram of protein for each pound of body weight. If you weigh 150 lbs, eat 150 grams a day. If you weigh 200 lbs, eat 200 grams of protein a day, and so on. Forget all the myths about kidney damage. Protein intakes at these levels do no harm to healthy kidneys. Even in your elder years, you can get stronger and bigger, but protein is the key. I weigh about 185 lbs but still shoot for 200 grams a day because it's easy for me to keep track of. At first, 200 grams seems like a lot. I'll teach you a few shortcuts to help get it done.

Whey protein (**wolfprotein.com**) is my main weapon of choice. I start my day with a scoop of whey in a glass of water or milk and I end my day the same way. Now we're at 40 grams. If I am struggling to meet my protein goal, sometimes I'll drink a cup of raw egg whites. Believe it or not, it has no taste. You just have to get used to the slimy texture. That is another 26 grams. Usually, at one point in the day, I'll eat a protein bar that ranges between 20-30 grams. You have to watch these as some of them are loaded with sugar. Remember to count your calories. A great healthy snack is a Greek yogurt. They contain usually 12-15 grams of protein per 150-gram cup. I love the ones from Chobani and it's not uncommon for me to have 2 cups a day. Cheese is another, a 1 ounce serving of cheddar cheese has 7 grams of protein. Almonds have 6 grams of protein per 1 ounce serving. Cottage cheese is loaded with protein with 1 cup having 25 grams. I list my favorite protein sources on a table in the Nuts and Bolts. (8)

Here's an example of how a non-workout day looks for me when I'm eating clean and getting ripped.

Food Intake	Calories	Protein
	Breakfast 7am:	
1/2 Cup of Oatmeal	150 Cal	5 Grams of Protein
2 Large Eggs	140 Cal	12 Grams of Protein
1 Scoop of Whey	130 Cal	20 Grams of Protein
	Snack 9:30am:	
Greek Yogurt	120 Cal	12 Grams of Protein
	Lunch 12pm:	
2 Cups of Salad with Low-fat Dressing	32 Cal	1 Gram of Protein
6 oz. Chicken Breast	260 Cal	52 Grams of Protein
	Snack 3pm:	
Protein Bar	300 Cal	30 Grams of Protein
	Dinner 6pm:	
6 oz. Turkey Breast	250 Cal	50 Grams of Protein
1 Cup of Green Beans	34 Cal	2 Grams of Protein
1 Cup of Cooked Carrots	82 Cal	1 Gram of Protein
	Snack 9pm:	
1 Scoop of Whey	130 Cal	20 Grams of Protein
12 oz. of Skim Milk	119 Cal	11 Grams of Protein
Totals:	**1747 Cal**	**211 Grams of Protein**

I'm to the point where I don't count calories too often because I know that if I'm eating fairly clean and I'm counting my protein, I'm going to be right around 2,000 calories. On the day of this chart, I got up at 6 a.m. and did 30 minutes on the elliptical trainer but lifted no weights. My fitness tracker band tells me I walked 12,095 steps, 5.61 miles and I burned 3,357 calories for the day. This keeps me at the goal of a 1,000 calorie deficit to maintain my weight loss of around .3 lbs a day. Technically, I had a net loss of 1,610 calories today, so I should have lost around .46 lbs of body fat. And I did – it's that easy!

Nuts and Bolts

(1) Here are a few suggestions I have regarding blood work. It's good to get a glucose test to see where your blood sugars are. There's the old standard, which is called a "fasting glucose test," and a newer, more effective test called the "HbA1c." I recommend getting an HbA1c test. The differences between these two tests are that the blood glucose test can be manipulated through diet and altered based on fasting times and other conditions. In other words, if you're behaving before getting your blood work, the test might give you results that are more favorable. The HbA1c test is more reliable in determining if you have an issue with blood sugar. The reason this is a very important test is because if your blood sugars are high, it greatly diminishes your metabolic ability to lose weight. I have seen many patients have their blood sugars corrected, and they lose 10 to 20 lbs without going on any diet.

It's a good idea to have your thyroid blood levels checked. The thyroid gland produces 2 hormones that greatly influence metabolic rate. If these hormones are out of balance you can eat like a bird and not lose any weight. If you need medication to correct abnormal levels of either of these hormones, a medical doctor can easily evaluate this and the cost of the medication is just pennies a day.

When doing blood work, it's also good to see what your lipids look like. I'd like to clear up a couple of misconceptions regarding cholesterol. Your total cholesterol is made up of LDLs, HDLs, and VLDLs. LDLs are low-density lipoproteins. VLDLs are very low-density lipoproteins. I like to think of low-density things like gum. Chewing gum has a low density, is very sticky, and binds to things easily. (I experimented with this phenomenon in the 1st grade with the bottom of my desk.) So if you have a lot of sticky lipoproteins in your bloodstream, they are more likely to stick to the walls of your arteries. On the other hand, HDLs are high-density lipoproteins. Think of high-density material as a metal BB. BBs don't stick to anything. They will just roll right off the table onto the floor. I would rather have my lipoproteins that are flowing through my arteries to be like BB's. Not only do these BB's not stick to the walls of the arteries, but some of the chewing gum on the walls of the arteries also comes off and sticks to the BB's, therefore cleaning the walls of the arteries. That is the beauty of good cholesterol!

Some people have high levels of HDLs that skew their total cholesterol levels. One thing that has driven me crazy about some general practitioners is that they see a person with a total cholesterol level of 220 and tell them they need to go on cholesterol-lowering medications. When looking at the cholesterol breakdown, their HDLs are 90, which gives them genetic protection from atherosclerosis. Would the general practitioner be happier if their HDL was 50 and now their total cholesterol would be 180?

Interestingly, women generally have better HDL levels than men. The higher our HDL levels, the better. Three ways to increase HDL is through aerobic exercise, fish oil intake, and mild alcohol consumption. Ideally, a woman's cholesterol HDL levels should be 65 mg/dl or higher; for men, 55 mg/dl or higher. A better way to calculate your cardiac risk is to look at your cholesterol-to-HDL ratio. Take your total cholesterol and divide it by your HDL. If your total cholesterol is 200 and your HDLs are 50, your cholesterol ratio would be 4 to 1. This is a good range, and any ratio below this number is better yet.

(2) The following is a chart listing many of the most common sauces, dressings, and condiments, along with their calories based on the volume of the serving. Remember, calories for most of the items that are shown are based on just 1 tablespoon. How many of us really use only 1 tablespoon? That's how diets get sabotaged.

Dressing or Sauce (1 tbsp)	Calories
Balsamic Vinaigrette	56
Barbecue Sauce	23
Béarnaise Sauce	62
Blue Cheese Dressing	80
Bolognese (Spaghetti Sauce)	240
Buttermilk Ranch Dressing	80
Caesar Dressing	64
Catalina Dressing	42
Chili Sauce	20
Cream Sauce	439
Curry Sauce	4
French Dressing	60
Gravy	123
Greek Dressing	70
Hollandaise Sauce	80

Dressing or Sauce (1 tbsp)	Calories
Honey Mustard Dressing	74
Horseradish	44
Italian Dressing	44
Ketchup	15
Mayonnaise	90
Mustard	3
Pesto	69
Ranch Dressing	77
Russian	60
Sesame Ginger Dressing	70
Sour Cream	26
Soy Sauce	10
Sweet and Sour Sauce	20
Tabasco	0
Teriyaki Sauce	16
Thai Curry Paste	23
Thousand Island Dressing	56
Tomato Paste	14
Tomato Sauce	59
Worcestershire Sauce	12
Zesty Italian Dressing	40

(3) Calories in various coffee products.

Beverage	Volume	Calories
Instant Coffee	8 oz.	4
Brewed Coffee with 2 tbsp of Cream	8 oz.	96
Brewed Coffee with 2 tbsp of Half and Half	8 oz.	37
Brewed Coffee with 2 tbsp of 2% Milk	8 oz.	15
Brewed Coffee with 2 tbsp of Powdered Non-Dairy Creamer	8 oz.	61
Brewed Coffee with 2 tbsp of Liquid Non-Dairy Creamer	8 oz.	37
Arby's Jamocha Swirl Shake	16 oz.	610
Dunkin' Donuts Brewed Coffee	10 oz.	15
Dunkin' Donuts Iced Coffee	16 oz.	10
McDonald's Brewed Coffee Large	16 oz.	0
McDonald's Latte	16 oz.	180
McDonald's Iced Coffee	16 oz.	280
Starbucks Brewed Coffee	16 oz.	5

(4) Adaptive thermogenesis is a medical term associated with extreme dieting causing the body to go into starvation mode. The body's innate intelligence has the ultimate goal of survival. We do not want to lower our caloric intake to such an extent that we force the body to function on fewer calories. This is where extreme low-calorie diets go wrong. We want to try to limit our calories, but not to the point where our bodies go into starvation mode. At the same time, we want to increase our caloric output through exercise to increase the metabolic rate. You can have it both ways here. Balance is the key. To prevent adaptive thermogenesis, a general rule of thumb is that women should not go below 1,200 calories a day and men should stay above 1,500 calories a day. If you go below 1,000 calories a day, I guarantee your body will go into starvation mode. Another unintended consequence is your body will start breaking down muscle to make sugar. We don't want to lose any muscle tissue. If you notice that you are getting close to the 1,000 calorie intake to facilitate the desired weight loss, I recommend increasing your caloric output by way of increased exercise. It's much better to burn the weight rather than starve it off.

(5) Many prescription medications can affect your body's ability to lose weight, both directly and indirectly, by increasing your appetite or limiting your activity level. Other medications directly affect your weight gains by increasing your water retention, like corticosteroids. A lot of antidepressants cause carb cravings and bloating. Some antipsychotic meds, antihypertensive meds, diabetes meds, and epilepsy meds can slow your metabolism. Even birth control pills have been known to cause weight gain. Simply enough, if you've started medicine and are gaining weight, consult your doctor.

(6) Here's a great table that lists the caloric values of some popular fruits and vegetables, which are a healthy source of carbohydrates.

Food	Quantity	Calories
Apple	1 Medium	65
Apple	1 Large	120
Apricot	1 Medium	100
Artichoke	1 Medium	20
Asparagus	6 Spears	20
Avocado	1 Medium	255
Banana	1 Medium	100
Banana	1 Large	120
Bell Pepper	1 Medium	30
Blackberries	1 Cup	50
Blueberries	1 Cup	80
Broccoli	1 Cup	20
Brussels Sprouts	4 Sprouts	25
Cabbage	1 Cup	20
Cantaloupe	1 Slice	55
Carrot	1 Medium	25
Celery	1 Stick	5
Cherries	1 Cup	100
Corn	1 Cob	155
Cucumber	1 Medium	45
Eggplant	1 Cup	20
Grapefruit	1 Medium	100
Grapes	1 Cup	60

Food	Quantity	Calories
Green Beans	1 Cup	30
Kale	1 Cup	35
Kiwi	1 Medium	40
Lettuce	1 Cup	5
Mango	1 Medium	150
Nectarine	1 Medium	60
Onions	1 Cup	45
Orange	1 Medium	80
Papaya	1 Medium	80
Peach	1 Medium	50
Pear	1 Medium	75
Peas	1 Cup	110
Pineapple	1 Cup	80
Plum	1 Medium	35
Potato	1 Medium	125
Radishes	1 Cup Sliced	19
Raspberries	1 Cup	65
Spinach	1 Cup	15
Strawberry	1 Large	10
Summer Squash	1 Medium	30
Sweet Potato	1 Medium	100
Tomato	1 Medium	20
Watermelon	1 Slice	70
Zucchini	1 Medium	30

Here's a list of my favorite protein-rich complex carbohydrates.

Food	Volume	Protein	Calories
Oats	1 Cup	13 g	303
Lentils	1 Cup	18 g	230
Quiona	1 Cup	8 g	222
Ezekiel Bread	1 Slice	4 g	80
Brussel Sprouts	1 Cup	4 g	56
Greek Yogurt	1 Cup	25 g	145
Sweet Potatoes	4 oz.	2 g	110
Green Beans	1 Cup	2 g	44
Rice	1 Cup	4 g	205
Broccoli	1 Cup	3 g	31

(7) My 10 favorite protein-rich fat sources.

Food	Volume	Protein	Calories
Almonds	1 oz.	6 g	161
Cashews	1 oz.	5 g	163
Peanuts	1 oz.	7 g	159
Pumpkin Seeds	1 oz.	5 g	125
Pistachios	1 oz.	6 g	158
Walnuts	1 oz.	4 g	183
Oysters	6 Medium-Size	8 g	175
Flax Seeds	1 oz.	5 g	148
Soybeans	1 oz.	10 g	50
Chia Seeds	1 oz.	4 g	101

(8) Here's a list of my 10 favorite protein sources.

Food	Volume	Protein	Calories
Chicken Breast	6 oz.	6 g	260
Turkey Breast	6 oz.	5 g	250
Egg	1 Egg	7 g	78
Tuna	1 Cup	5 g	179
Whey Protein	1 Scoop	6 g	130
Fresh Fish	6 oz.	4 g	250
Shrimp	6 oz.	8 g	168
Lean Beef	6 oz.	5 g	368
Scallops	6 oz.	34 g	180
Beef Jerky	1 oz.	4 g	116

CHAPTER TWO

Supplements

Vitamins, Minerals, and Supplements – The Real Truth

The vitamin section of this book could be an entire text in itself. As a chiropractor, I found myself to be the target of every herb and vitamin salesman out there. I wanted all of these things to work but found very few things were what they were cracked up to be. On the other hand, vitamin, mineral, and herb supplementation can be a natural way of healing.

Not all vitamins, herbs, and supplements are needed. Sometimes, financial profits can be more of a motivation to the one selling vitamins than the health results for the customer. So, if a salesman tries to sell you something and what he says doesn't make a lot of sense, don't be surprised. I remember a vitamin salesman telling me about this strange, detoxifying herb that I had never heard of. I asked him, "How does it work?" He replied that he wasn't sure and that he's not a doctor but he knows that after taking these herbs his feces smelled awful. He concluded the smell was toxins being eliminated from his body. I explained to him that he was eating something that wasn't needed in his body and that the material was putrefying in his intestines and therefore creating the horrible smell. For the purposes of this book, I am going to try to keep it simple and tell it how it is...which leads to our first lesson on vitamins.

A) Vitamins

Vitamins are compounds that are needed for normal cell function. There are two types of classifications for vitamins. One is essential and the other is nonessential. There are thirteen of them. Eleven essential vitamins are not produced in the body and must be taken in by way of food sources. These are vitamin A, B1, B2, B3, B5, B6, B9, B12, C, E, and lastly, K. There are two nonessential vitamins, meaning that the body can synthesize them on its own. These are vitamin D and vitamin B7, more commonly known as Biotin. In the Nuts and Bolts section of this chapter, we will put a list of foods where these vitamins are found, and also conditions that can result from deficiencies thereof. (1)

B) Minerals

Essential minerals are elements that our body needs for normal cellular activity from muscle contraction, nervous system function, and general fluid balance. These minerals include calcium, chloride, iron, magnesium, phosphorus, potassium, and sodium. These elements are responsible for so many different vital functions.

I'm a big believer in taking a multivitamin daily. It makes sense and it's an efficient way to get some of these nutrients. Most multivitamins should have the essential vitamins, and the minerals calcium, magnesium, and zinc. Additionally, there are usually trace minerals like copper, chromium, iodine, and selenium. If you're doing a lot of exercising, you should add extra calcium, magnesium, and potassium supplementation, as these three electrolytes play a vital role in electroconductivity of the nervous and muscle tissue. If you are someone who doesn't want to take several vitamins, I recommend at least taking a multivitamin. I have come up with a multivitamin that helps with the needs of both men and women (**wolfmultivit.com**).

Remember, vitamins and minerals play a role in cellular functions just as motor oil plays a vital role in keeping the engine of your car from failing. Vitamins and minerals don't do anything for energy, just as motor oil doesn't make your car go faster. Carbs and fats are your body's analog to gasoline in your car. So, if you're taking vitamins you won't necessarily experience any boost in energy. That doesn't mean they are not important for your health, and it makes complete sense to take them.

You might ask, "What additional vitamins should I take?" A proper diet should include foods that are high in most minerals and vitamins that your body needs. That said, we all have genetic predispositions for certain illnesses. I find it useful to look at your family history and see if there's a clear predisposition for a certain illness. For example, my family has issues with congestive heart failure, so it makes sense for me to throw in a couple of extra nutrients that help with functions of the myocardium of the heart. I take coenzyme Q10 (**wolfcoq10.com**) a magnesium mineral supplement (**wolfmegamag.com**), and Omega 3 fish oils. (**wolfomega3.com**) Most vitamins are water-soluble, meaning if you take too much, basically you have expensive urine. However, you must be careful with the fat-soluble vitamins – being vitamin A, D, E, and K – because they are stored in the liver and the body's fatty tissues. When taken in excess, they can create damage. With the exception of vitamin D, I don't recommend taking any of these in supplemental form in amounts larger than those found in a multivitamin. Usually, we get enough in our diet. If you want to take vitamin A, I recommend taking beta-carotene instead, because your body will only break down the amount of vitamin A from beta-carotene that it needs. Regarding vitamin D, I recommend getting blood work to determine if you need to take it in supplemental form. Instead of critiquing each vitamin, herbal, and mineral supplement separately, I am going to include a comprehensive table noting the effectiveness of a particular supplement. I am going to give each supplement a one- to four-star rating based on my personal and clinical experience. This list can be found in the Nuts and Bolts section of this chapter. (2)

C) Herbs

Herbs are plant substances that have different mixtures of chemicals that can be used to treat medical conditions. For those that question the usefulness of plant compounds for their healing properties, let's break it down into simple terms. Pharmaceutical agents are refined chemical compounds that interact with our body chemistry to effect changes. Most of the drugs manufactured worldwide have plant derivatives. These drugs are used to facilitate a specific response. It's just chemistry, nothing magical. The same holds true for herbal compounds. They are chemical agents that can affect the physiology of our bodies. Herbal medicines can be much more affordable and easier to obtain. The benefits of botanical medicines are unquestioned. I have noticed clinically many herbal products work well when placed in combination with another herb. For example, when it comes to fighting inflammation, turmeric works better with ginger. (**wolftumeric.com**) The same principle holds true with prescription medication. An example of this on most prescription medicine bottles is the warning label which states, "do not consume alcohol while taking this drug." This is because the chemical compound – alcohol, in this instance – can enhance the chemical property of the drug and act as an accelerant to the prescription medication. We can use these accelerants to our advantage with certain herb combinations. In the Nuts and Bolts section of this chapter, I'll list some of the best herbs – and their benefits – that might be worth trying. (3)

D) Sports Supplements

There are a lot of sports supplements out there and sometimes making the right choice can be confusing. There are a couple of mainstay amino acids that you can't go wrong with. Additionally, we will talk about pre-workout drinks and supplements.

1) Creatine

Creatine is king because it works. Creatine is found in meats. However, it makes more sense to take it in supplemental form because of such low concentrations in meat products. There has been a lot written, both good and bad, on creatine. In my experience the only true concern with taking this supplement would be if you had an underlying kidney disease, or if you are taking any medication that creates stress on the kidneys. If so, consult your primary care physician before taking the supplement. I've been taking creatine for 15 years with no ill effects. Also, I found that you do not need to do any "loading phases." (By this, I mean taking a higher dose the first few days.) I take a 5 gram scoop of creatine monohydrate before I workout and 5 gram scoop of creatine monohydrate (**wolfcreatine.com**) in my post-workout shake. You will notice the difference right away! One of the initial negatives of taking the supplement is that you will retain a little water. That's because muscle tissue is mostly water. It enhances the ability of your body to grow muscle. So initially, there will be a small weight gain due to increased muscle mass and increase water retention in muscle tissue. There are many different types of creatine compounds, of which I have tried several. Many are expensive and have no additional benefits. Creatine monohydrate works just as good as any of them. I have not noticed any difference in performance taking the other creatine compounds. I recommend just getting a big jar of the powder and mixing the recommended amount with your shakes. It's very affordable and incredibly effective.

2) BCAAs

Another popular muscle building supplement is branched chain amino acids. Basically, the three amino acids – isoleucine, leucine, and valine – are the BCAAs. Leucine is the one I've noticed that makes a difference. A lot of protein powders and some protein bars put BCAAs in their formulas. Leucine is the one that I use as part of my pre- and post-workout drink. I buy a big jar of it and take 1 scoop containing 5 grams before and after working out. The one thing you need to know about this supplement is that it does not mix well with every kind of drink. A shaker bottle does not cut it. You will have to get a blender and mix it that way. Another great time to take BCAAs is at night before you go to bed for maximum muscle recovery and optimal gains. (**wolfbcaa.com**) Check out our website at **DrDeanWolf.com** for a great video showing how easy it is to mix and make protein shakes.

3) Glutamine

Glutamine is another amino acid that I use. All the research on glutamine seems to point to the fact that it helps with muscle recovery more than it does with muscle building. I can't say that I found a great amount of gains with this amino acid. I take it because the research shows that it does help with some recovery. As we get older, we need all the help we can get. I take Glutamine which is found in my night time recovery BCAA supplement. (**wolfbcaa.com**)

4) Pre-workout Drinks

What are pre-workout drinks? These drinks give you more energy and help with a more complete workout. I have tried several pre-workout drinks and I have to admit I do love these. My favorite is the one I developed called Nitric Shock Pre-Workout Body Boost. (**wolfnitricshock.com**) One common denominator of all these drinks is that they contain caffeine, and there's a good reason for that. Caffeine helps you with mental focus and acuity and gives you an increased energy level that you need for a good workout. Caffeine is known to boost your metabolism, which helps you burn more fat. With workout drinks I like to have beta-alanine, which helps you with fatigue and cellular stress. Another is citrulline malate, which helps increase blood flow and anaerobic energy. You'll find a little creatine in the mixture as well. These pre-workout drinks aid in the growth and development of muscles by helping carbs, fats, and protein metabolize properly. I feel like my workouts are more complete. However, you have to consider the cardiac risk if you're taking caffeine and some of these compounds, coupled with raising your heart rate by lifting weights or doing aerobic training. If you are going to take any of these pre-workout drinks, get a check-up by your doctor to see if your heart is strong enough. It might be a good idea to get a stress test to see what your cardiovascular conditioning level is. Discuss this with your doctor. Once you've developed some cardiac endurance and have been cleared by your health care professional, you can have at it. Now that we know what to eat and what to take, let's get mean and lean!

E) Joint Supplements

As we age, joint degeneration is inevitable. Taking joint supplements can help relieve pain and slow the degenerative process. With such a large selection of joint supplements on the market, making the right choice of which ones to take can be difficult. There is so much conflicting information but I have found there are a few time-tested compounds that work very well.

The first one I recommend is glucosamine sulfate. When you go to the vitamin store and look at the joint supplements available you might notice that almost everyone has glucosamine in them. Not every item has chondroitin, MSM or SAMe. That's because glucosamine works. I've had a lot of clinical experience with great results with glucosamine sulfate. The glucosamine hydrochloride is not as effective. Additionally, I have found MSM and chondroitin not to be very effective on their own. In combination with glucosamine they are very productive. I recommend taking 10mg of glucosamine sulfate (**wolfjointrebuild.com**) per pound of body weight per day. So, if you weigh 150 pounds take 1,500mg/day. If you have a shellfish allergy you might want to avoid taking glucosamine because a lot of the glucosamine supplements are derived from shellfish.

My second recommendation is Type II collagen. Type I and Type III collagen are good for your skin, nails, and hair. Type II is the protein that helps cartilage and joints. It's worth noting that it's been found to be more effective taking the Type II version without Type I and III present for better absorption. Additionally, it's been shown that vitamin C helps enhance the absorption of Type II collagen. I recommend taking the hydrolyzed form of Type II collagen with your morning drink. I get this supplement in powder form in a 1 kilogram bag. Take a tablespoon a day.

Lastly, I recommend taking tumeric with ginger. This is another example of two different supplements that act as accelerants with one another to help reduce inflammation in the joints (**wolftumeric.com**). I recommend taking 1,000mg/day of turmeric and 200mg/day of ginger. Turmeric can interact with a few stomach medications. So, if you take some meds for stomach issues, check with your doctor or pharmacist to see if there are any contraindications.

Nuts and Bolts

(1) This table shows a list of foods for the 13 vitamins we need and where to find them. Also, their functions in a healthy body and disorders from deficiencies thereof.

Vitamins	Where to find	Role in the body	Associated disorders due to deficiency of this vitamin
Vitamin A	Liver, Cheese, Eggs, and Carrots	Important for vision, immune function, and reproductive health	Hair loss, vision problems, and susceptibility to infections
Vitamin B1	Pork, Legumes, Nuts, Seeds, Fortified Cereals, and Fortified Grains	Important for maintaining healthy metabolism, digestion, and nerve function	Nervous system diseases, fatigue, forgetfulness, and gastrointestinal disorders
Vitamin B2	Fortified Cereals, Fortified Grains, Lean Meat, Poultry, and Dairy Products	Important for energy metabolism. Helps adrenal function and supports normal vision and healthy skin	Eye disorders, inflammation of the mouth, and skin issues
Vitamin B3	Lean Meats, Seafood, Eggs, Legumes, Milk, Breads, and Cereals	Very important for energy metabolism and growth	Memory disorders, dementia, depression, and fatigue
Vitamin B5	Almost all foods contain vitamin B5	Helps control blood sugars and metabolism	Fatigue, headache, nausea, and tingling in the hands
Vitamin B6	Meat, Fish, Poultry, Grains, Cereals, Green Leafy Vegetables, and Soybeans	Important for nerve and red cell blood function, promotes protein and carbohydrate metabolism	Anemia, headaches, nausea, and flaky skin
Vitamin B7	Egg Yolks, Soybeans, Whole Grains, and Nuts	Important for healthy metabolism	Anemia, depression, hair loss, and high blood sugar
Vitamin B9	Green Leafy Vegetables, Asparagus, Orange Juice, Avocados, Legumes, and Fortified Flour	Helps with the production of DNA and RNA, synthesizes certain amino acids which is helpful in pregnancies	Birth defects, anemia, digestive disorders, and fatigue

Vitamins	Where to find	Role in the body	Associated disorders due to deficiency of this vitamin
Vitamin B12	Found in All Animal Products	Very important for nerve function and DNA and RNA synthesis	Bone loss, fatigue, depression, and digestive disorders
Vitamin C	Found in Most Fruits and Vegetables	Important in the body for repair and growth	Scurvy, bleeding gums, and susceptibility to infection
Vitamin D	Seafood, Eggs, Milk, and Exposure to the Sun	Necessary for calcium absorption and bone growth	Rickets and osteamalacia
Vitamin E	Avocados, Cold-Pressed Vegetable Oils, and Green Vegetables	Prevention of cell damage and helps the immune system	Damage to blood cells and nervous system tissue
Vitamin K	Broccoli, Brussel Sprouts, Cauliflower, and Green Leafy Vegetables	Extemely important in the process of blood clotting	Problems with insulin release and glucose regulation

(2) The following tables are compilations of vitamin, mineral, and herbal supplements, respectively. I include the more common vitamins, minerals, and herbal supplements. These supplements are rated from one to four stars. If it's not on this list, chances are it's not even a one-star rating in my book and not worth taking. One star means you really don't need to buy this product to take in supplemental form unless it matches up to specific illness or needs unique to you that could benefit from the additional nutrition. One thing to keep in mind, some one- or two-star rated items work to a three- or four-star performance when combined with other one- or two-star elements. If any item is listed in these tables, I think it has some value. Two-star rating means it's okay in some circumstances to take in addition to a well-rounded diet but most often not necessary. Three stars mean this is a good one to take with little or no downsides.

Four-star rating means this is the real deal. I would recommend these to anyone for overall positive benefits.

Vitamin	Rating
A	*
B Complex	***
B1	***
B2	***
B3	***
B5	*
B6	***
B7 Biotin	***
B9 Folic Acid	* (**** for pregnant women)
B12	**
C	**
D	**
E	*
K	*
Multivitamin	****

Minerals	Rating
Calcium	***
Chromium	*
Copper	*
Iodine	*
Iron	* for men *** for women
Magnesium	****
Potassium	***
Selenium	*
Zinc	**

Sports Supplements	Rating
Arginine	* Do not take if you take lysine
BCAA's Together	****
Caffeine	***
Casein Protein	*
Creatine	****
Glutamine	***
Isoleucine	***
Leucine	***
Lysine	*
L-Tyrosine	*
NO2 or other pre-workout drinks	****
Valine	***
Whey Protein	****

(3) Herbs and Miscellaneous Nutritional Products and Associated Health Benefits

Herbs/ Nutritional Products	Rating	Health Benefits
Alfalfa	*	Alfalfa is a natural herb good for bladder, kidney, and prostate conditions. It has been shown to have benefits against high cholesterol, diabetes, rheumatoid arthritis, and asthma. It is a great source of Vitamins A, C, E, and K4. It may also aid in the fight against high cholesterol and diabetes.
Ashwagandha	**	This herb has been shown to help lower cortisol levels in individuals that often suffer from high levels of stress and depression. Overall, it's helpful with many other body functions, such as reducing heart disease risk, decreasing cholesterol, and increasing brain function.
Buckthorn	*	Sea buckthorn oil comes from sea buckthorn fruit. The oil from this fruit is rich in vitamins and nutrients. Since this compound reduces platelet aggregation, it's useful in helping prevent blood clots.
Cat's Claw	*	Cat's Claw is a vine that is found in the Amazon rainforest and other tropical locations. It's known for anti-aging nutrients. Chemicals from this plant have been found to have anti-inflammatory effects, as well as immune system boosting functions and gastrointestinal benefits.
Cayenne Pepper	*	Cayenne peppers contain capsaicin, an active component that helps to boost your metabolism. It helps by increasing the body temperature and, in doing so, causes the body to burn more calories per day. This process is known as diet-induced thermogenesis, which causes an increase in your metabolism.
Chamomile	**	This herb's abilities have been well documented and proven to be a strong contender in helping with sleep and relaxing nerves. There have also been studies that have shown chamomile to have other benefits, such as anti-inflammatory effects.

Herbs/ Nutritional Products	Rating	Health Benefits
Chondroitin Sulfate	*	Chondroitin Sulfate is found in most cartilaginous tissues in our body. In supplemental form by itself, it hasn't been found to be effective. However, when combined with Glucosamine Sulfate, studies have shown it can aid in joint repair
CoQ10	****	Commonly used for helping heart issues, this compound can be effective for conditions such as heart failure, chest pain, and high blood pressure. CoQ10 could even improve symptoms and decrease the risk of a future cardiac issue. It also lowers blood pressure. This is the real deal and one of my personal favorites. Everyone not taking blood thinners should take Coq10.
DHEA	*	DHEA is often referred to as "the mother hormone." Important hormones such as testosterone and estrogen are derived from DHEA. Because higher hormone levels can help reduce fat, DHEA has been found to aid in dieting, as well as appetite suppression.
Echinacea	*	Echinacea is a North American plant which has many chemical compounds that have been known to boost immune system function. This one is a good one to take if you get sick.
GABA	*	GABA is a naturally occurring acid within the central nervous system of humans. It's the primary neurotransmitter inhibitor, in charge of reducing excitability in neurons. Some studies have shown that people with high stress and/or depression tend to have lower naturally occurring GABA molecules in their body.
Garcinia Cambogia	**	Garcinia supplements come from the peel of the fruit Garcinia Cambogia. High amounts of HCA are found in the extracts. HCA can contribute to weight loss.

Herbs and Miscellaneous Nutritional Products and Associated Health Benefits continued...

Garlic	**	Garlic is much more than just a flavor in your meal. It has hidden health benefits you might want to consider. This type of onion is high in Vitamin C, B6, and manganese. By adding garlic to your diet, you could reduce the likelihood of catching the common cold or the flu.
Ginger	**	Ginger is a natural anti-inflammatory and a strong antioxidant.
Ginkgo Biloba	**	Gingko plants are loaded with antioxidants. Therefore, it is useful in preventing cell damage, which can decrease the likelihood of cancer. It's been known to aid vascular problems, which, in turn, can aid sexual energy. Another common boast is its ability to help with cognitive functions of the brain.
Ginseng	**	Like Gingko, Ginseng has high amounts of antioxidants, which may help decrease potential cell damage. Its vascular benefits include increased sexual function and better blood circulation. Ginseng has been known to increase energy levels and fight fatigue.
Glucosamine Sulfate	***	Glucosamine has been around for a while because it works. It helps with degenerative changes in joint cartilage. The sulfate version of Glucosamine is more effective than with the hydrochloride component. Also, Studies have shown that it works well with Chondroitin and MSM.
Goldenseal	*	This plant found in the northeast United States has been used to treat a variety of conditions. Its most notable benefit is how it may aid in digestive functions. It works well with echinacea.
Grape Seed Extract	*	Some studies have shown there are wonderful benefits from using grape seed extract. It has been used for a number of cardiovascular conditions and poor circulation of the veins. It could also lower cholesterol.
Green Tea Extract	**	Common to the East, this extract has proven great for sustaining health. Loaded with polyphenol antioxidants, it reduces inflammation, boosts metabolism, and sometimes even accelerates fat loss.

Herbs and Miscellaneous Nutritional Products and Associated Health Benefits continued...

Hawthorn Berry	*	There is a reason these berries are known as the "cure for a broken heart." They help with anxiety and depression. The whole plant is used to make medicine. It is also used in support of helping heart health, controlling high blood pressure, and high cholesterol.
Horny Goat Weed	**	More scientifically known as Epimedium, some studies show there are several benefits of this plant. Its properties could help keep bones strong, protect nerves, and support the immune system. It has been beneficial for those with erectile dysfunction.
Lactobacillus Acidophilus	**	Lactobacillus Acidophilus is a bacteria found in your intestines. This bacteria is key for normal digestion. If you have any digestive issues, this supplement can help. Also, this is a must after any trial of oral antibiotic therapy.
Melatonin	*	This hormone is produced in our brain. Its role in aiding restful sleep has been well documented. Since there is no rebound effect, it's safe to take.
Milk Thistle	*	Milk Thistle is most known for its role in liver support.
MSM	**	MSM's claim to fame is joint support. This one works well with glucosamine.
Omega 3 Fish Oil	***	Omega 3's are a combination of EPA and DHA. This helps to maintain a healthy heart and blood system, and reduces the risk of developing heart disease or having a stroke. These risks are reduced by preventing arteries from clogging, chest pain, irregular heartbeat, heart failure, and blood clots.
Passion Flower	*	Passion Flower has been known to help with anxiety. This is another herb that works better in combination with other compounds.
Probiotics	***	Probiotics help with bacterial flora in our digestive tract. These are great to use after any antibiotic treatment.
Red Yeast Rice	*	This is the product of yeast grown from white rice. This compound has the same ingredient found in the prescription drug Lovastatin. Red Yeast Rice is a natural statin and lowers cholesterol.

Herbs and Miscellaneous Nutritional Products and Associated Health Benefits continued...

Saw Palmetto	*	This plant is native to Malaysia (South East Asia). It is a shrub that appears similar to a small tree. In Malaysian culture, they used the root of the plant as a medicine for centuries. Some studies have shown that it's an effective energy booster, fat burner, and testosterone regulator.
Spirulina	*	Naturally found as an algae, Spirulina had been used in the herbal practice of Aztecs for centuries. Modern medicine has rediscovered it and researched its many benefits. Packed full of nutritional value, this "superfood" has been known to support metabolism and reduce heart health problems.
St. John's Wort	**	This herb is another good one. It clearly helps with depression. The only concern with St. John's Wort is that it has numerous side effects when taken in combination with prescription drugs.
Turmeric	**	Turmeric is the spice that makes curry yellow. It has a powerful, anti-inflammatory effect and is a strong antioxidant. Its main component curcumin is more effective than many prescription anti-inflammatory drugs. Turmeric works well with ginger to help with joint pain.
Type II Collagen	****	Collagen is the main component of the cartilage in the joints of our body. Type II collagen is responsible for the tensile resilience of the joint cartilage. For degenerative joint disease, this one works better than Type I or Type III.
Turmeric with Ginger	***	These two play well together. This should be in everyone's daily arsenal who suffer from any inflammatory disorders.
Valerian	*	This herb helps promote falling asleep. It works well with other sleep agent herbs.

CHAPTER THREE

Orthotics

A) Orthotics are the Secret to Foundational Health

It all starts with the feet. Our feet are the platforms of our bodies. It's paramount to your structural health to have your foundation on level ground, especially if you are going to do any type of aerobic or weight training. If the bricks at the bottom of a building are not situated correctly, the bricks at the top of the building will be leaning even more. Not to mention, problems with the feet can manifest themselves in the form of knee, hip, and back pain. When working out, you geometrically increase the likelihood of these medical conditions if your feet aren't on even ground.

B) Pronation is Problem Number One

A normal healthy foot has a nice arch. When the structures that maintain the arch of our foot fail, the arch collapses. You have probably heard the familiar term "flat feet." This condition can be congenital. Some individuals are born with it and other times it's acquired from injury or excess mechanical stress. When the arch collapses, pronation of the foot occurs. This happens to 80% of the population.

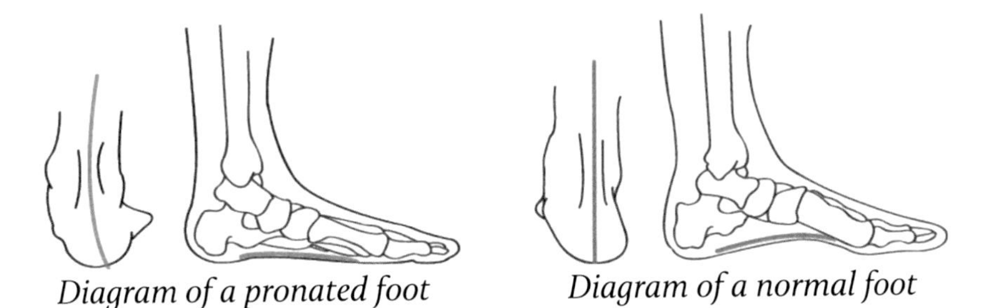

Diagram of a pronated foot *Diagram of a normal foot*

As we age, the soft tissue components of the foot lose their resilience. This loss of integrity causes the foot to pronate and the arch collapses. Pay close attention to the following diagram. It shows how pronation of one foot can simply wreak havoc on the mechanics of the entire body. In this example, pronation of the foot on the left creates a little torque on the Achilles tendon and causes internal rotation of the tibia and femur, resulting in a varus formation of the knee. The hip is now lowered on that side, increasing the stress placed on the hip joint. This lowered hip results in a compensatory lumbar scoliosis, which in turn drops the shoulder on the opposite side. As a result, the head tilts and the neck turns.

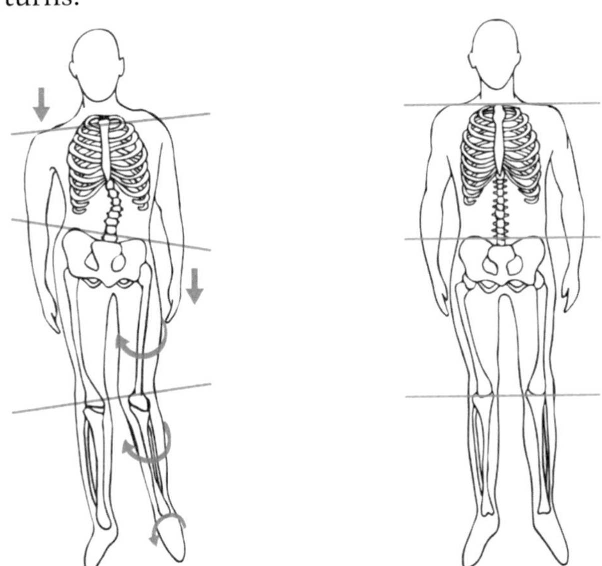

Diagram of kinetic chain with foot pronation and without

Just imagine the extra stress a pronated foot puts onto the Achilles tendon while doing a leg press or running. Or how about the extra pressure exerted onto the knee with the same activities? The hip joint and low back can also be the target of injury from collapsed arches.

C) Orthotics

An orthotic is a simple appliance that is placed under the foot to aid in the stability of the arch. Everyone should wear orthotics, particularly when participating in any aerobic activity or weight training. They can be made of plastic or leather, and I've even seen them made of metal. The most important feature of an orthotic is functionality. It must work! You cannot have a flimsy piece of foam and expect it to support the weight of your entire body. I am amazed at how much junk is offered on the market today. I purchased the first ten orthotics I found online, and I could collapse the arch completely with a few pounds of pressure from my fingers on every single one of them.

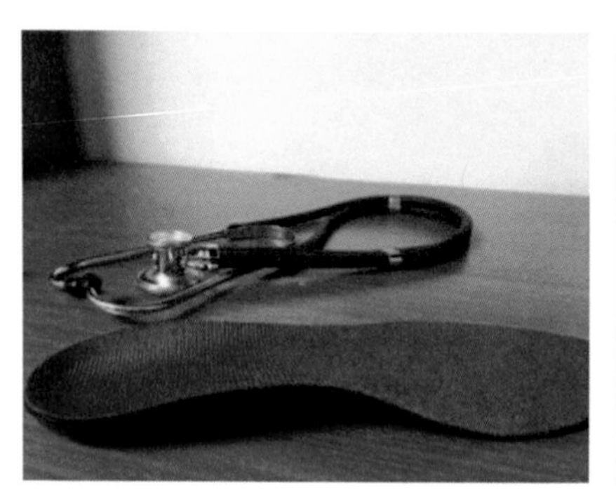

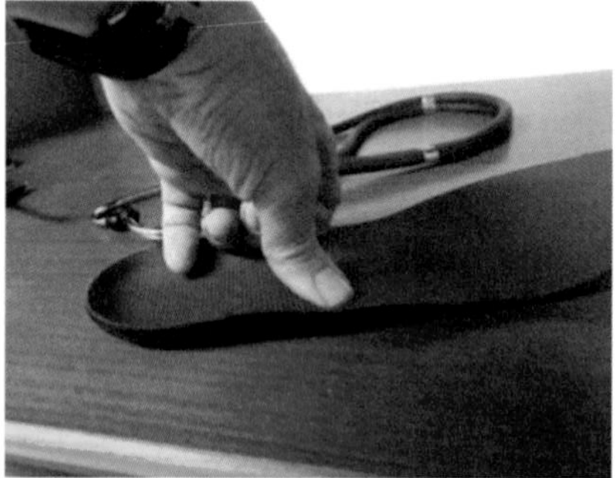

Imagine the weight of your entire body on the device. Wearing that type of insert is pointless. The following picture shows the difference in arch structure with the cheap orthotic, on the left, and a good orthotic on the right. What a difference in mechanical support!

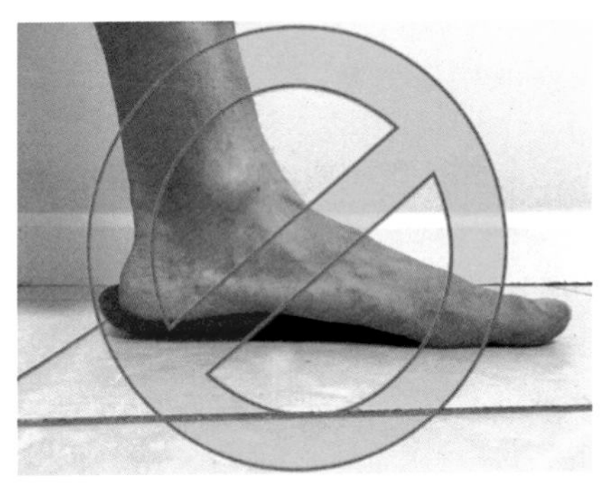
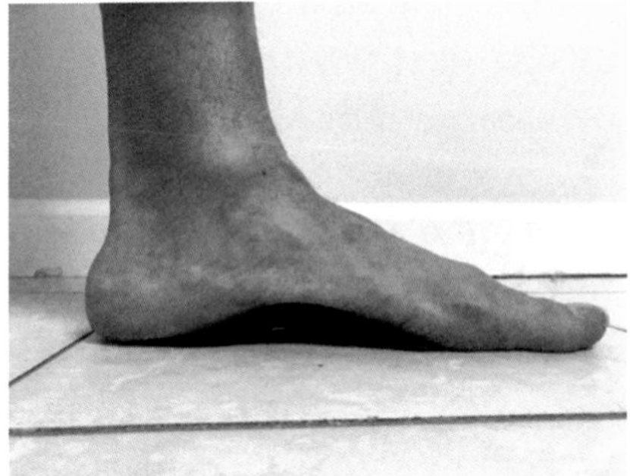

1)The doctor conspiracy

Often times, a doctor diagnoses the patient with a disorder that would be corrected by orthotics. Their first plan of action is to then recommend a cheap alternative to expensive "custom made" orthotics. They will sell or recommend flimsy foam foot inserts that functionally don't work. They look nice, they are soft and comfortable, but they are ineffective. They charge twenty or thirty dollars for equipment that will fail. Thus, there's another follow-up visit to the doctor with another office visit fee, yet the patient still has foot pain. The doctor claims to have tried the conservative route, but now justifies the need to make a custom orthotic. A custom orthotic could cost a few hundred dollars. The orthotic is so effective and delivers results. So, most patients are happy to fork over the cash, even though it costs more. Fortunately, there is an effective and affordable alternative. I designed an orthotic that works the best – at one-tenth of the cost of the "custom made" orthotics.

2) Are they really custom?

I made "custom" orthotics for dozens of companies. I was always in search of the perfect orthotic that had a price point within reason. I went through the routine of molding the patient's foot, measuring, and making notes of any anomalies. I would then package the mold and send it off to the lab, only to get the orthotic back a week or two later and find they all looked the same. I guess rightfully so. The basic idea is to put a foundation under the arch of the foot to support the foot in the most optimal mechanical position. I started questioning how "custom" these orthotics really were. I read a few research papers which stated that a well-made, hundred dollar arch support that is sturdy can be as good as a custom orthotic – the keyword being "sturdy." The orthotic must be firm. It must brace the foot and arch and hold it in the proper position. Previously, I had made leather orthotics that were pretty firm and thought they might have had a softer feel. However, the leather would degrade over time and then we'd have to make another orthotic. There goes another couple hundred dollars. Leather material is not cost-effective.

3) How hard should an orthotic be?

I worked tirelessly trying to come up with the right material combination. Then, I came across a type of blended plastic that I could heat in an oven, allowing me to shape it easily. When heated, the plastic became soft and I could mold the orthotic into any position I wanted. Surprisingly, I found that the hard firm orthotic felt soft in a soft shoe and felt firmer in a dress shoe. Regardless of the type of shoe, this orthotic worked. The orthotic plays an intimate role in the foot's support, so the shoe dictates the comfort. In any case, the orthotic must be sturdy to keep the arch from collapsing.

4) How thick should the orthotic be?

After researching different designs, I created a perfect orthotic that functionally supports the foot in the best position. Many of the existing orthotics were so cumbersome that, in order for it to fit, the inside of the shoe had to be ripped apart. I was motivated to create a sleek, yet durable material. I wanted the orthotic to be as thin as a dime. The idea was to design an orthotic that didn't require a person to do anything other than slide the orthotic immediately into their shoe. I have done just that! Remember when I mentioned that there was an effective and affordable alternative? This orthotic is superior in so many ways. The material is light, durable, and thin enough to fit into any shoe without modification.

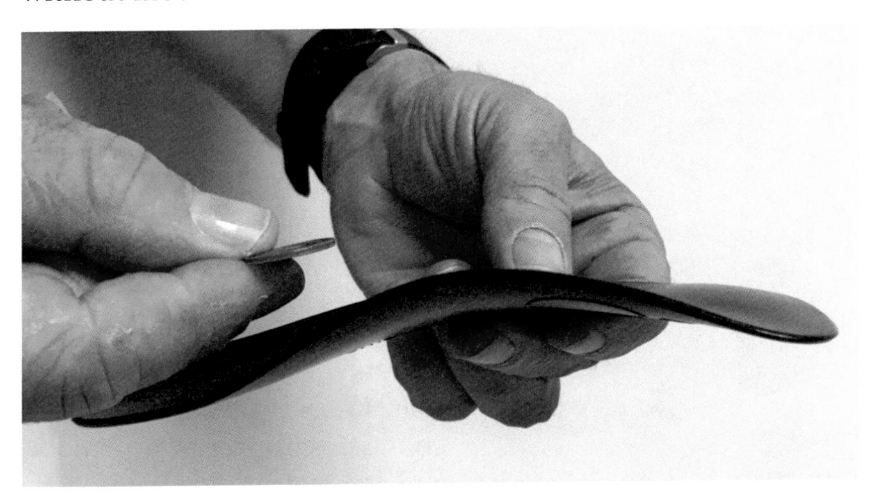

Furthermore, since they do not break, they don't need to be replaced later. Wolf Orthotics are not only highly functional, they are the most cost effective alternative as well. (**wolforthotics.com**)

5) How long should the orthotic be?

Another thing I experimented with was the length of the orthotic. I've found that the longer the orthotic, the more problems fitting the apparatus into a shoe. Additionally, the difference in the sizes of our feet primarily comes from the difference in the lengths of the metatarsal and phalangeal bones. The arch of the foot is made up of the metatarsal and tarsal bones. This is where the orthotic functional zone needs to be to get the job done. By making the orthotic ¾ length, instead of the entire length of the foot, it eliminates variability in shoe sizes from one foot to another. In other words, if one foot was a half size larger or more than the opposite foot, two different sizes wouldn't be necessary. Additionally, the three-quarter length orthotic is easier to fit into any shoe.

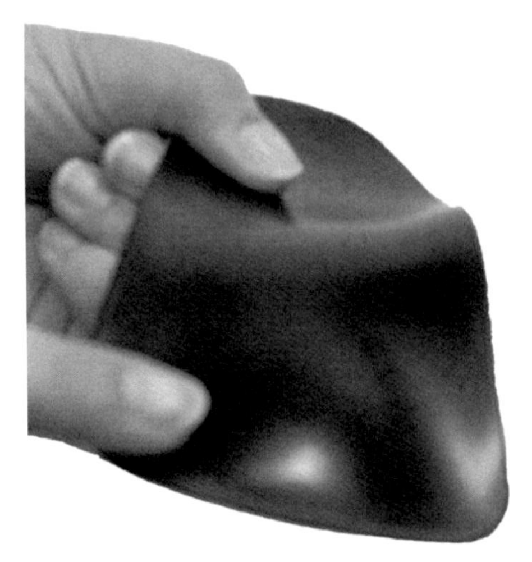

6) Spread out

I found that putting a little bump at the end of the orthotic (where the metatarsals start) helps to slightly spread the toes apart, making for better balance and eliminating other potential foot problems caused by toe crowding. This is very useful during exercise and competition. I highly recommend that you visit my website, **DrDeanWolf.com**, and check out my orthotic. This orthotic is simply the best and completely affordable.

7) Break-in period

The one complication when using an orthotic for the first time is the potential for a needed break-in period. Clinically, I have found about 30% of my patients need a brief break-in period. If you put the orthotic in your shoe and find your arch to be a little sore after about an hour, simply remove the orthotic for an hour. Then, reinsert it in your shoe for another hour. After another hour, take it out for an hour. Repeat this process for just 1-2 days. It takes a relatively short time for your foot to get used to the arch support. Usually, after 1 day the opposite effect will occur. Your foot gets accustomed to the proper support of the orthotic and you won't want to be without it.

One last thought. Even if your feet have no loss of arch, you will benefit by wearing orthotics. Orthotics will keep your arch from flattening and keep the foot in the optimal position for strength and performance. Helping maintain this position prevents injuries from ever occurring.

The Nuts and Bolts section of this chapter will deal with specific foot disorders that are cured by simply wearing orthotics. If you have no problems with your feet, you can fast forward to the next chapter.

Nuts and Bolts

1) *Plantar Fasciitis*

Pronation of the foot causes so many mechanical failures in the foot itself. When the arch collapses, the bottom of the foot has an excess traction load. This traction load pulls on the plantar tendon and stretches the plantar fascia.

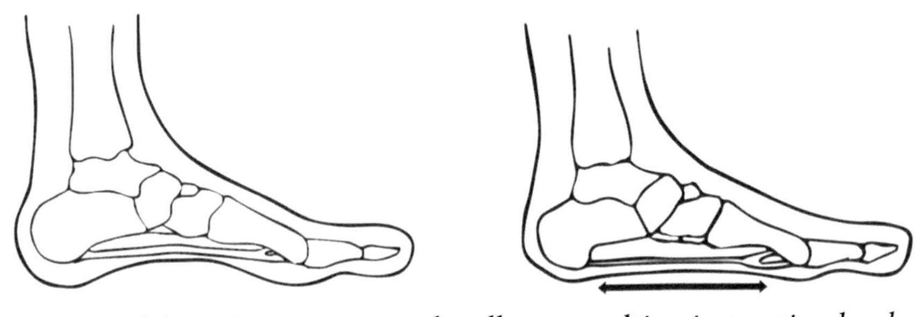

Normal foot view *Arch collapse resulting in traction load*

Excess traction creates microscopic tears in the tendons and fascia. Then, the tissue contracts and shortens. This condition is called plantar fasciitis. Typically, a person suffering from plantar fasciitis will experience a lot of pain in the bottom of the foot as soon as they get on their feet after rest. When sleeping or resting, the fascia contracts from the excess traction load that was induced by microtrauma experienced earlier in the day. The body tries to heal all those microscopic tears. These little scabs, if you will, form in an effort to patch things up. Arising after rest, the arch collapses, thereby pulling on the fascia again and ripping all the scar tissue apart. Hence, the pain in the morning when putting weight on the feet.

This process is what makes you feel like you're 100 years old when taking your first few steps in the morning. Even sitting down at lunch for 15 minutes will be enough time for the plantar fascia to contract, resulting in pain in the bottom of the foot when standing up. Most of us will have pronation issues as we get older. Even with the healthiest individuals, the plantar fascia loses its elasticity and resilience with age. Anyone that gets out of bed with discomfort in the bottom of the foot is suffering from plantar fasciitis. An orthotic will eliminate this pain completely in a relatively short period of time. (**wolforthotics.com**) If you are in the acute phase of plantar fasciitis go to my website **DrDeanWolf.com** to view a video that demonstrates a taping procedure that can help reduce some pain from this condition.

2) Plantar Fascia Tear

If you tear the plantar fascia, you will experience severe pain in the bottom of the foot. This pain will temporarily make it practically impossible to walk. When tearing the plantar fascia, taping will help tremendously in managing the pain and restoring function. Orthotics are a must in this situation. If you have a plantar fascia tear, go to my website **DrDeanWolf.com** and watch the video demonstrating a taping procedure that can alleviate pain from this condition.

3) Heel Spurs

There's a law of physiology called "Wolff's Law." (No relation to the author.) It states that bone increases density proportionally to the amount of stress placed on the bone. All of our bones have little spurs which serve as anchor points for the tendon to insert into the bone. If there is an increase in demand at these anchor points, the body has to build a bigger anchor to avoid rupture of the tendon insertion. This is how a forensic pathologist can dig up the remains of a body that's hundreds of years old and make a model of exactly how he or she looked. If a man has 18-inch biceps, the spurs or anchor points that glue the bicipital tendon into the bone are much bigger than a man with 12-inch biceps. The same principle holds true for the plantar tendons of the foot. The plantar tendons are used to flex the toes. We use this grasping movement of the toes when we walk. When the arch collapses, this puts an extra strain on the anchor point in the heel. As a result, the body increases the spur or anchor to accommodate the extra force placed on it.

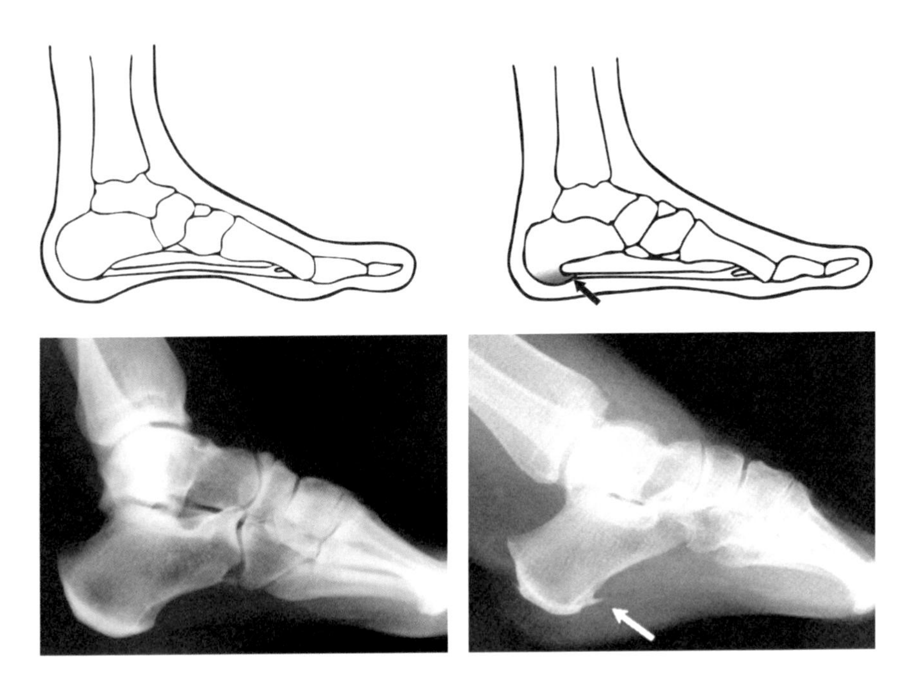

This phenomenon is no problem when we make our biceps bigger. The problem with our feet is that we walk on them. Making a bone point on a heel bigger, longer, and sharper presents an entirely different dynamic. A lot of doctors treat heel spurs with cortisone shots and stretching routines. The cortisone helps with inflammation and the stretches temporarily alleviate some fascial contractures. However, the fundamental problem is that the arch is collapsing. Stop the arch from collapsing and the pain will stop. Orthotics can fix this in a short period of time. (**wolforthotics.com**)

4) Achilles Tendinitis

Achilles tendinitis is a potentially serious condition. It's usually caused by pronation of the foot. When the foot pronates, the Achilles tendon bows. The bowing effect creates a lot of stress on the tendon and its insertions. If untreated, the tendon may rupture. This is a great way to get an ambulance ride to the hospital. Inflammation can be treated with anti-inflammatory medications, ultrasound therapy, and a lot of ice and stretching. Most importantly, stop the pronation from occurring with an orthotic. (**wolforthotics.com**) Orthotics fix this problem by eliminating bowing of the Achilles tendon.

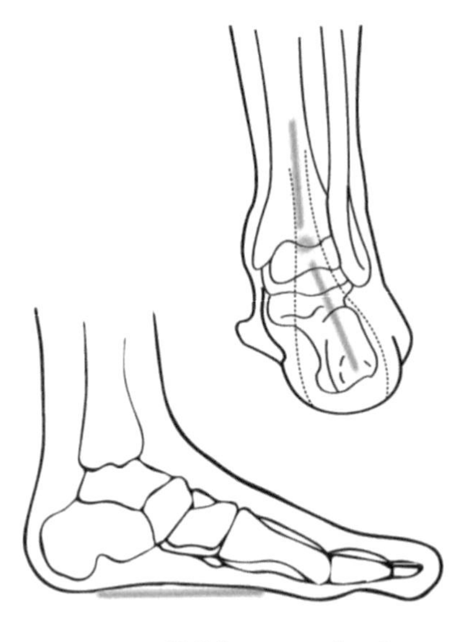

Without orthotic

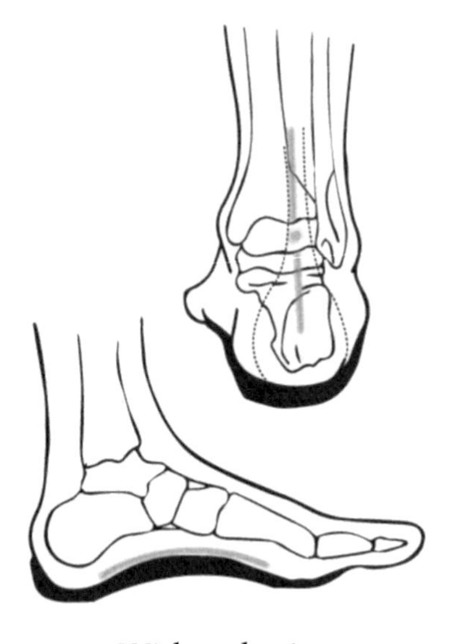

With orthotic

CHAPTER FOUR

The Cause of Joint Pain

A) Joint Translation

In this chapter, we're going to discuss joint translation. The purpose of this book is to teach you how to get in great shape in your 40s, 50s, and beyond. With that in mind, I felt it important to discuss joint translation and give you an understanding of how injuries occur before we discuss exercising strategies. In medical texts, joint translation is referred to as: *laxity, looseness, glide, hypermobility, instability, multidirectional instability, or Joint Hypermobility Syndrome,* just to name a few. I might use some of these terms interchangeably, but I like to call these joint problems "translation." In this chapter, I'm going to explain exactly what translation is, identify the root cause, and how to recognize it. Most importantly, I will also explain how to guard against translation, and what you can do about translation issues.

Let's start by defining joint translation. To fully understand, we're going to review some of the basic anatomy of a joint. Anatomically speaking, a joint is the point where two bones in the body meet.

The joint helps accommodate movement of the two bones. As shown in the diagram below, a joint is made up of cartilage and a capsule containing a membrane with fluid. This fluid acts like oil for smooth joint motion. Additionally, we have tendons and ligaments. A tendon is tissue that connects the muscle to a bone, and a *ligament* is tissue that connects one bone to another bone in the joint.

NORMAL JOINT

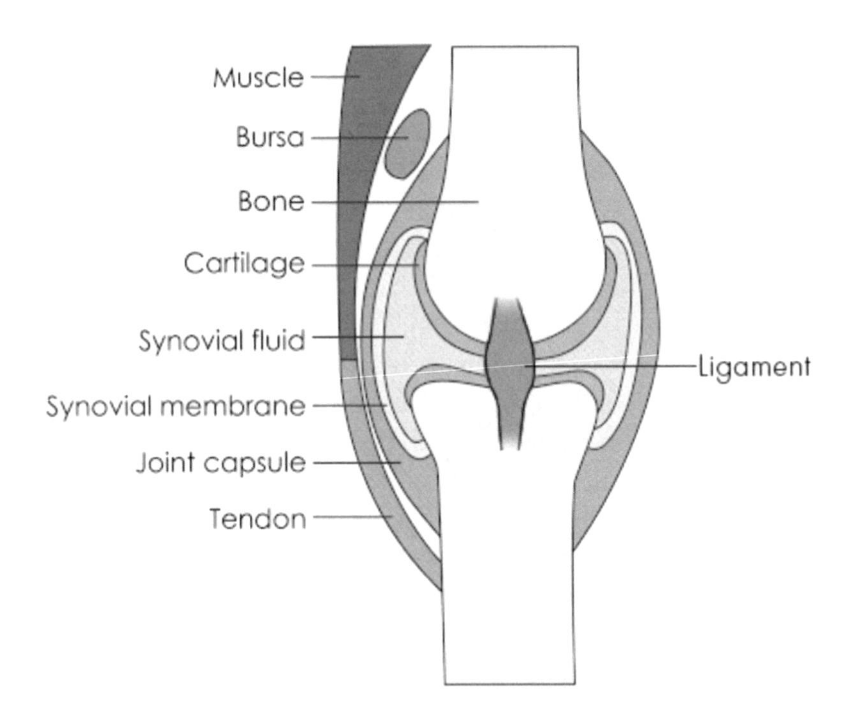

It's very important to note that ligaments are the **primary** stabilizers of a joint, meaning that ligaments are the number one way our bodies hold one bone to another. The **secondary** method of stabilization in our body is through muscles. Muscles help the ligaments hold the bones together. A tendon connects the muscle to the bone. When there is an injury to the ligaments, the muscles play a more important role in stabilizing the joint. Because of added stress on the muscle, both the muscle and tendon are now vulnerable to injury.

Technically, there are numerous joint classifications, including structural classifications and biomechanical classifications. We have ball-and-socket joints, such as those in the hips and shoulders. There are condyloid joints in the wrist. Hinge joints are found in the elbow and knee. Gliding joints also known as cartilaginous joints that are located in the vertebral column. The thumb has a saddle joint. There's even a pivot joint found in the neck. Lastly, there are immovable joints like the suture joints of the bones of the skull. For simplicity's sake, we are going to discuss the most common joints and problems associated with joint translation.

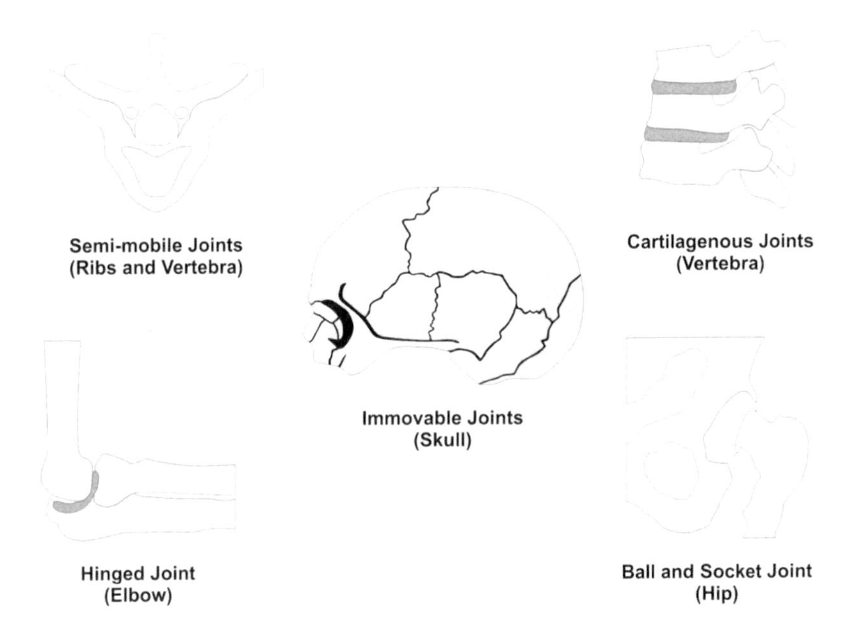

Joints that are movable function in a set range of motion. When the joint moves **outside of its normal range of motion** – a range that it is not supposed to be moving into – that is called *translation*.

Joint translation causes problems. When a joint translates, there is a shear created in the wall of the joints from movement or grinding. This creates microtrauma to the capsule of the joint. I like the word microtrauma because it accurately describes what happens, meaning it hurts the joint a little bit, and then a little bit more, and then a little bit more, until little tears appear in the connective tissue. Then, inflammation occurs and the baroreceptors (pressure receptors) of the joint send a message to the brain saying there is achiness or pain. Another consequence of microtrauma is that cumulative trauma can cause the complete tear of a structure by a seemingly innocuous event. Many patients seen in my office will say something like, “I just threw the dog a bone and I felt this sharp pain in my shoulder.” The last throw was the straw that broke the proverbial camel’s back. Or in this instance, a complete tear of the rotator cuff. This is the end result of chronic translation.

In most cases, patients I’ve treated can’t recall a specific injury. They usually relate that their back “just started hurting.” This is because they have been suffering chronic microtrauma from translation deformities that are finally causing joint injury. Get it?

When translation occurs in joints, it can affect athletic performance. For example, have you ever wondered why a pitcher in Major League Baseball can throw the ball 90 miles an hour but the average man cannot? Some of these players look like they weigh 160 lbs and wouldn’t be too useful in a barroom brawl. Or have you ever wondered why some people are so much better than others at arm wrestling? It all comes down to capsule strength and stability. The less a joint translates, the greater the mechanical advantage. Think of it like this: If you are trying to move a boulder with a crowbar, you need a fulcrum to increase your mechanical advantage. You might use a smaller rock as a fulcrum to pry the boulder from its position.

The small rock must not move (translate) so that you have a mechanical advantage.

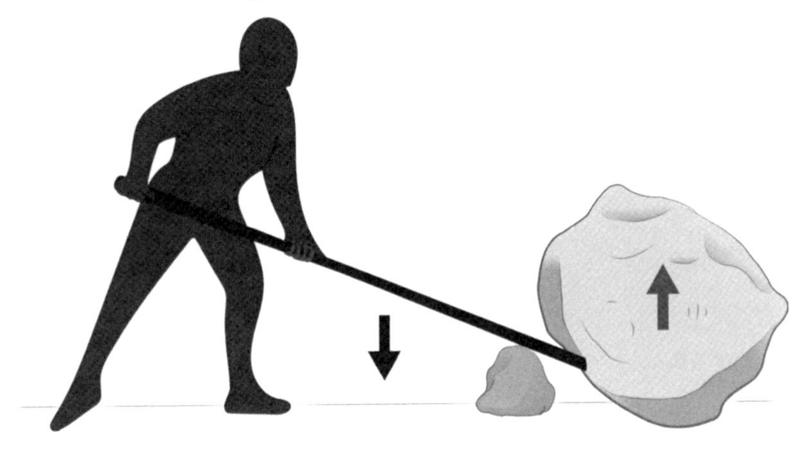

What if you used a piece of softwood as the fulcrum? As you pry, the wood deforms – "translates" – and the boulder will not move.

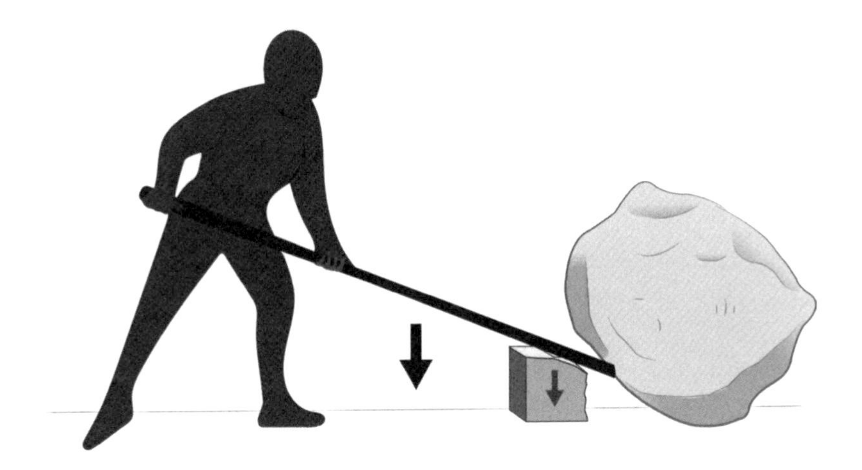

Typically, professional athletes are signed to big contracts pending a physical. Translation deformity is what the sports physicians are looking for. For example, if a pitcher has a lot of instability (translation) in their shoulder, it's only a matter of time before a muscle is injured trying to help stabilize the shoulder. That's what rotator cuff injuries are all about. If a football player has a lot of looseness (translation) in his knee, odds are he's going to tear some cartilage or a ligament from a big hit sooner than later.

B) Four Major Causes of Translation

There are four major causes of joint instability. The first one is congenital, meaning that a person was born with a lot of movement in the joint. The second major cause is overuse. The third is blunt trauma from an accident or fall. The fourth cause is degenerative joint changes that occur as we all get older.

1) Congential

Congenital joint translation is very common. Have you ever seen someone with bad posture? Usually, a person with poor posture has primary posterior instability (looseness) of the shoulder joint. The back of the shoulder is not held tight by the ligament. It could be a function of congenital agenesis (a missing ligament),or because the ligament or capsule is not very tight. This results in the physical appearance of the person having drooping shoulders or their shoulders appear to be rolled forward. Eventually, a person with this condition will hurt their shoulder throwing an object. This is a very common presentation in young adults and is a leading cause of rotator cuff injuries.

Have you ever heard of someone that is double-jointed? Guess what? This is a person that has congenital joint translation deformities. The reason a person can subluxate (dislocate) some of his joints is because there is an excess amount of laxity usually due to a ligment agenesis (missing), or extremely loose ligaments resulting in hypermobility (excess movement) of the joint capsule. There's actually some good news with this group of people. In their geriatric years, they will have a better range of motion. As we get older all of our tissues get stiffer and harder, resulting in less motion. As long as there's not a lot of trauma to the joint from injury, people with joint translation fare pretty well with the amount of motion they have in their senior years.

2) Overuse

The second major cause of joint translation is overuse. In Major League Baseball, they have determined that each pitcher has only so many fastballs in them. That is why they pay a lot of attention to pitch counts. No matter how strong a player is, if the joint is overused, microtrauma occurs to the stabilizing tissues, resulting in looseness, or laxity of the joint. This damage could be to the cartilage of the joint or it can be to the actual capsule. This also places excessive stress on the tendons and ligaments of the joint, resulting in injury. Microtrauma can occur in everyday life. A carpenter swinging a hammer, a factory worker repetitively pushing or pulling all day long, and delivery people that get in and out of their vehicle hundreds of times a day can all suffer microtrauma and subsequent injury to joints over time.

3) Trauma

The third major cause of joint translation is trauma to the joint. Obviously, if someone falls off a ladder and dislocates his shoulder, there is going to be some form of joint injury. Most severe traumatic joint injuries result in some form of permanent damage with resulting chronic translation issues.

4) Degenerative Disease

Last but not least, there is degenerative joint disease (DJD). Degenerative joint disease is also known as osteoarthritis and is, in fact, the most common form of arthritis. This happens in all joints, including the spinal joints. Degenerative disc disease (DDD) occurs in the spine as well. This section might get a little technical. I'm going to explain what happens when we get older and why we get injured.

Unfortunately, degeneration takes place in all of our joints as we age, resulting in some form of translation. This degeneration occurs primarily due to dehydration of our tissues. In the spine, the discs function as cushions between the vertebrae, playing an important role in stability of the spine. They act like glue between the vertebrae.

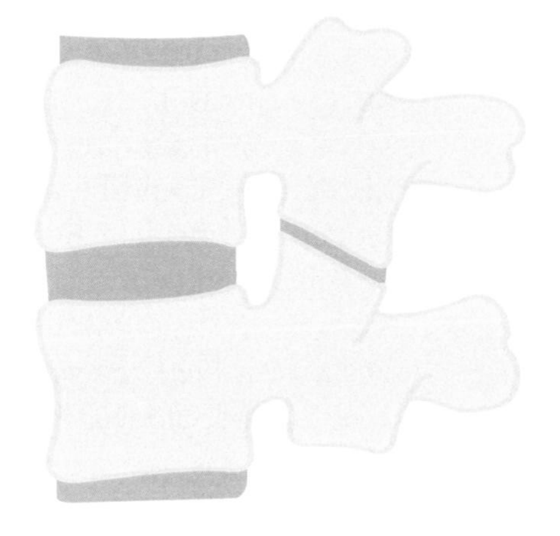

When dehydration of the disc occurs, spacing and stability are lost. The joints in the back of the spine lose water, too. As the following image shows, when the disc degenerates and loses height, the joint itself becomes loose.

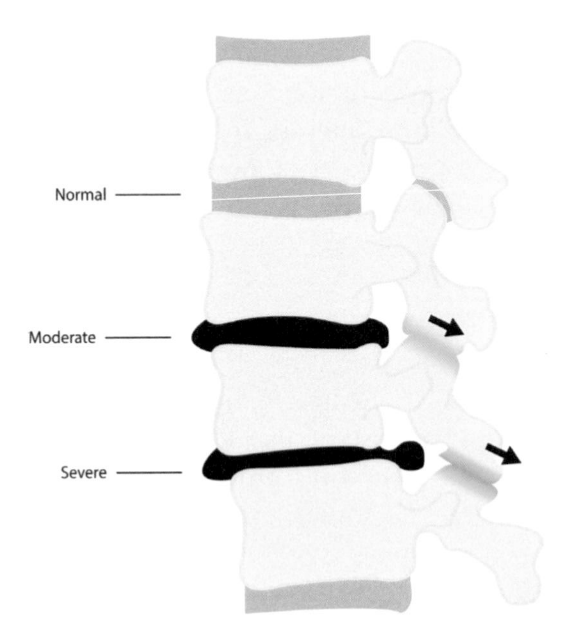

The loss of disc stability forces more pressure on the joints in the back of the spine – the facet joints. Then, posterior translation of the joint occurs. And with translation, there is further damage to the joint and disc. It becomes a domino effect.

C) Magnetic Resonance Imaging (MRI)

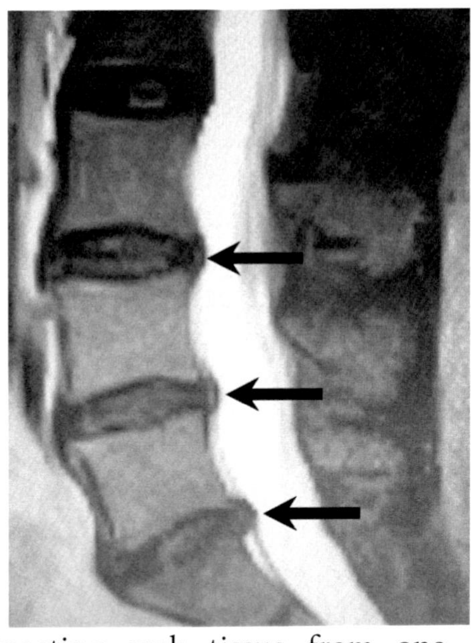

Basically, an MRI is a giant magnet. When you get into an MRI machine, a magnetic field goes through your body. Hydrogen is a positive ion (H+) and is found in water. Good old H2O. A giant magnet tilts elemental hydrogen on its axis, allowing the scanner to produce an image based on the amount of hydrogen something has. The more water in tissue, the brighter the image. Since each of our body tissues contains different concentrations of water, delineating each tissue from one another, a beautiful image can be created. A healthy disc is white. A diseased disc is black and here's why. As we age, the soft tissues lose water concentration and become brittle. On an MRI, these tissues now start to look black or gray because of less water. In 30 years of practice, every herniated disc I have ever seen is black on MRI.

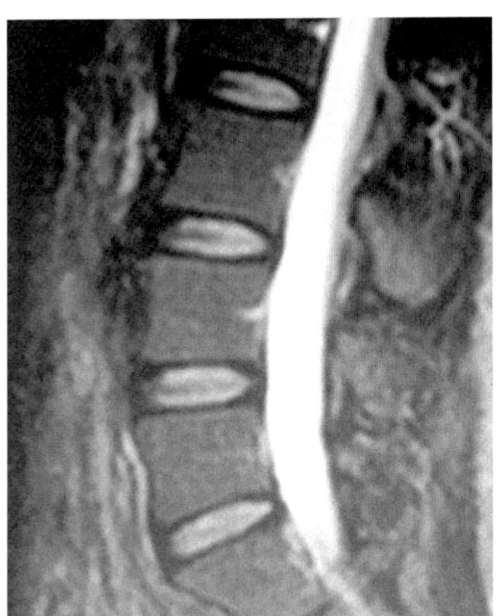

Every healthy disc is white, meaning there is a lot of water content.

A healthy disc is extremely strong like all fibrocartilage; e.g., the labrum (cartilage on the joint socket rim) of the hips and shoulders and the meniscus of the knees. In young people, this tissue is extremely hard to tear under normal circumstances.

Think of the connective tissue in our body as being like a rubber band. A brand new rubber band is very resilient and can be stretched easily. Take a rubber band that's been sitting in a drawer for 2 years and stretch it and see what happens. It's likely it will break. With the old rubber band, you can see the dehydration and you can feel the different texture. This is a great example of what happens with the degeneration phase of aging and how it affects the soft tissues of our body. This process starts to occur in our late 20s and early-30s. A prime example is an NFL running back. Take a 24 year-old running back and a 34 year-old running back and have them remove their shirts. They both look like action figure dolls. Both are completely ripped and in great physical shape. However, when the 24 year-old running back gets hit, he bounces up off the turf like nothing happened. The 34 year-old running back gets injured. The 44 year-old weekend warrior gets hurt at the gym lifting something he's lifted a thousand times before without incident. The 54 year-old gets injured after bending over to tie his shoes. The 64 year-old gets injured and doesn't even know what he did. So on and so forth. The more we age, the more brittle the tissues get.

If you have a recurring injury, you probably have a form of joint translation. For example, if you have noticed that you continually get a stiff neck, you probably have a translation deformity at one or more of the motor units of the cervical spine. If you have noticed that you have stiffness in your knees after walking on the treadmill or jogging, you probably have joint translation issues with your knees. If your back "goes out" 1-2 times a year, you probably have laxity in one or more of the joints in your back or hip that predisposes you to this injury. If you notice your shoulder is always sore after you hit a large bucket of golf balls, you probably have a joint translation problem.

In the Nuts and Bolts section of this chapter, we are going to discuss the mechanisms behind the most common joint translation problems. I will label each section according to the body part that is injured. That way, if you don't have that particular problem, you can move onto the next chapter. Later in this book, I will go into greater detail as I teach you how to compensate for these issues, as well as how to properly train to strengthen the joint through alternative methods. Having joint hypermobility issues is not the end of the world. Following my tips, you can greatly reduce chronic pain and increase the quality of your life.

Nuts and Bolts

1) Shoulder

Let's start with the shoulder joint. Typically, this joint will translate the most while still being functional. When doing the simple act of an arm curl with weights, a healthy shoulder joint stabilizes the *humerus* (the bone in the upper arm) as shown in the picture below.

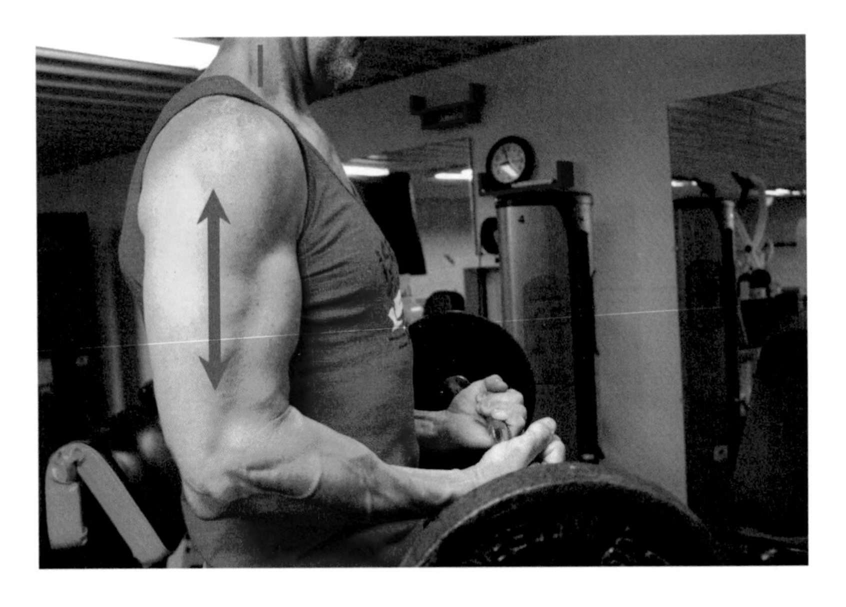

When translation occurs, the *humeral head* (the top part of the upper arm bone) will move *anterior* (forward) in the joint, creating a decreased lever and causing friction inside the joint as shown in the following picture. Some textbooks call this "anterior humeral glide." As you can see from the following picture, my shoulder wants to move up and forward when I do a curling motion.

I am a perfect example of what a translation deformity looks like.

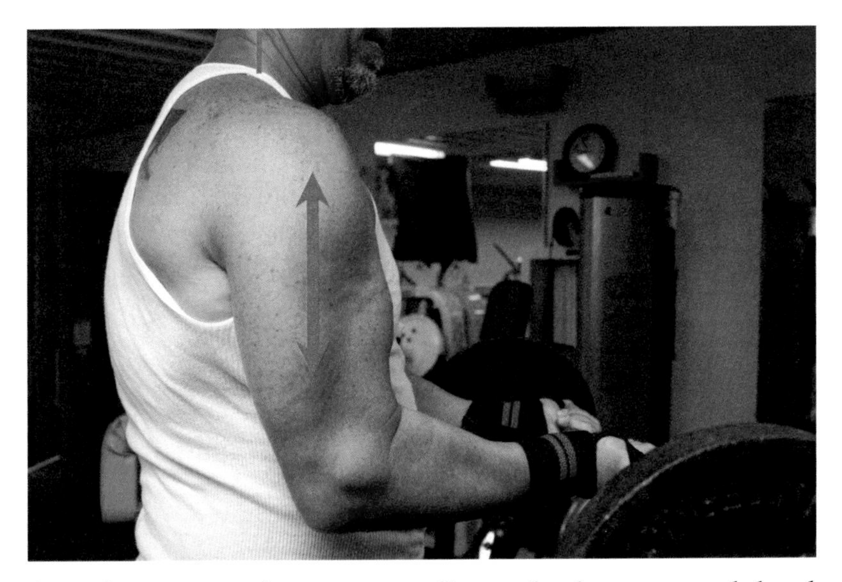

When this occurs, the rotator cuff muscles have to work harder to hold the bones in place, predisposing one to cuff injury. Additionally, more stress is placed on the cartilage lining the joint, which results in labral trauma. The best way to avoid injury while doing a curl is to hold the elbows back when lifting the weight. Lift the bar up in a curling motion never allowing the bar to leave the front of your body. This minimizes translation and protects the shoulder from injury. The picture to the right shows how great this position accomplishes reduction in shoulder translation.

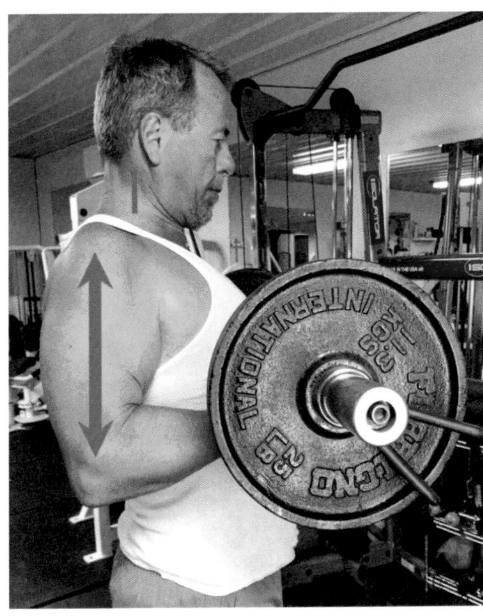

There can also be both anterior and posterior translation deformities of the shoulder. The best way to counteract instability issues of the shoulder is to strengthen the secondary stabilizers of the shoulder. Do you remember when we discussed primary and secondary stabilizers earlier in this chapter? Muscles are always secondary stabilizers of joints. You will hear a lot of this in the remainder of this book. Secondary stabilizers are the secret to managing primary stabilizer deficits. Anytime there is a translation deformity, we are going to work on the muscles that surround the affected joint. This concept is the keystone to most physical therapy programs. In the shoulder, the rotator cuff muscles are the secondary stabilizers of the shoulder.

The rotator cuff is a group of four muscles that encapsulate the top of the humerus. These four muscles control all internal, external, and abduction motions of the arm.

Rotator Cuff Muscles

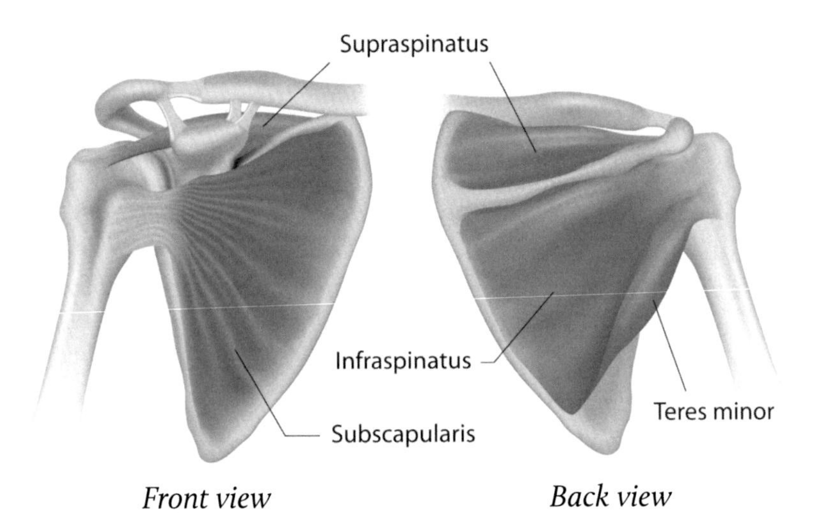

Front view *Back view*

Generally speaking, the infraspinatus and teres minor work together to create external rotation of the arm. The subscapularis internally rotates the arm. The supraspinatus abducts the arm. I have found that subscapularis injuries are rare. Typically, I have my patients refrain from working internal rotation exercises. There are exceptions. If there's clearly damage to the subscapularis and no damage to the cartilage, exercises would be appropriate. However, if there is a translation deformity of the shoulder, internal rotation typically magnifies anterior glide and creates a little shear to the labrum (cartilage on the shoulder socket rim), thereby exacerbating the laxity of the shoulder and harming the articular cartilage.

You can work the cuff with as little as two exercises. I love to use exercise resistance bands for these routines. You can easily put the bands in your pocket and you don't need any gym equipment. (**wolfbands.com**)

For the first exercise, I recommend doing an abduction motion only to 45° while making sure that the thumb is pointing down to isolate the correct muscle. It's the same position as pouring water out of a glass.

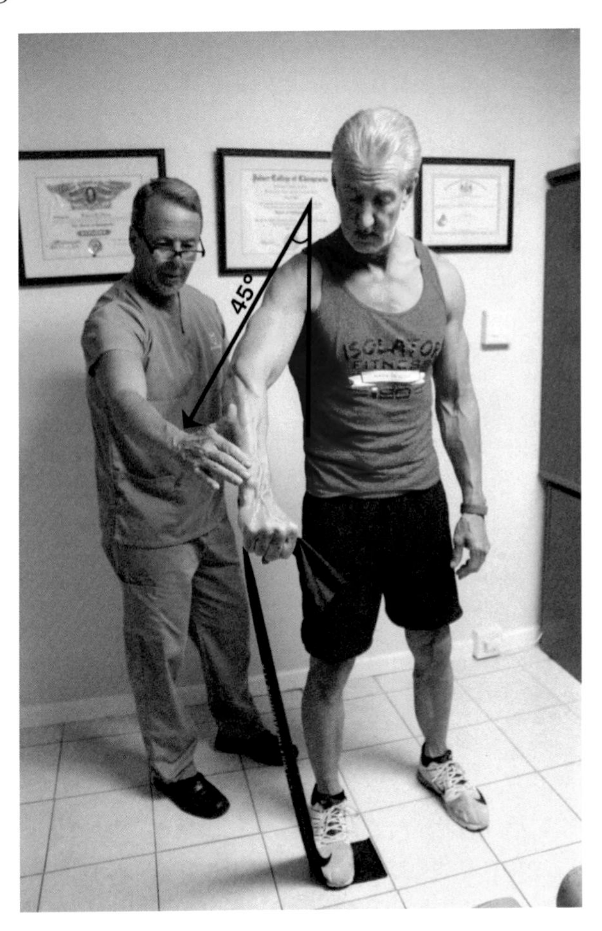

When researching for this book, I was amazed at how many images and YouTube videos show people performing these exercises incorrectly. The following picture demonstrates the incorrect way to exercise the supraspinatus muscle.

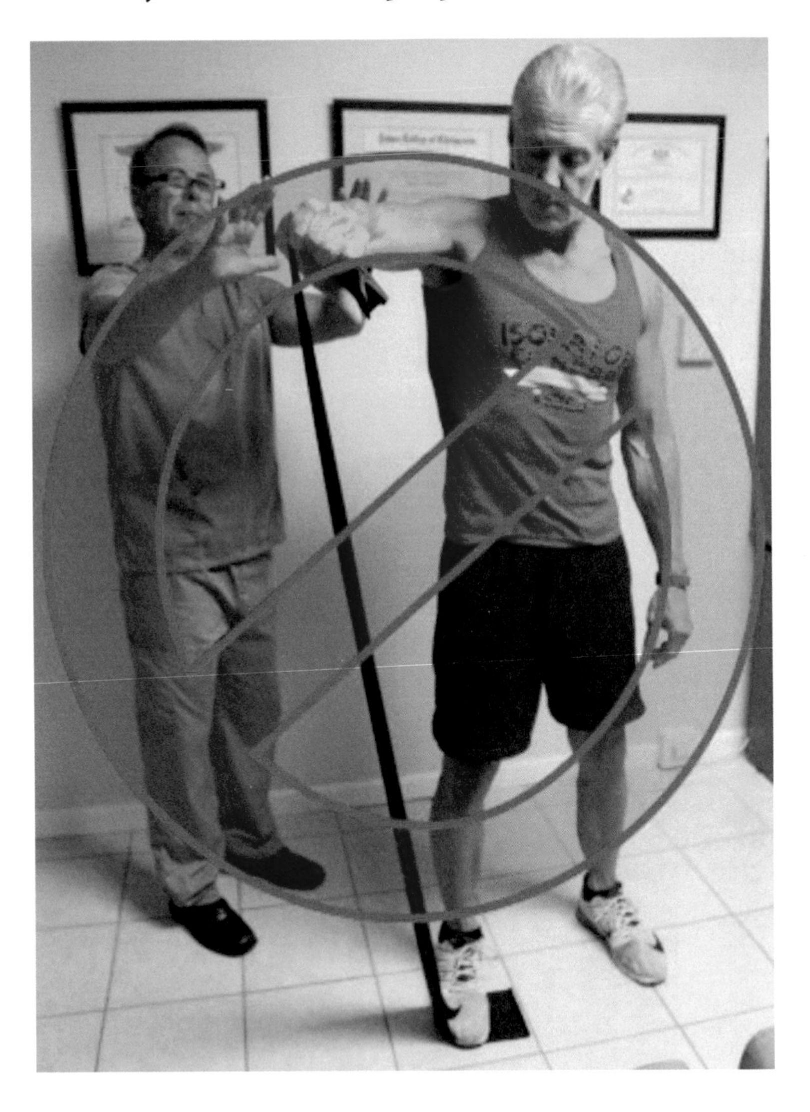

Never go higher than 45° because the wrong muscle group will be worked. Improper form can irritate the shoulder by creating impingement, which I discuss in the shoulder section of Chapter 9.

For the second exercise, I recommend doing an external rotation movement. Start with one hand against the stomach with your elbow fixed at your side and then rotate 90° outward.

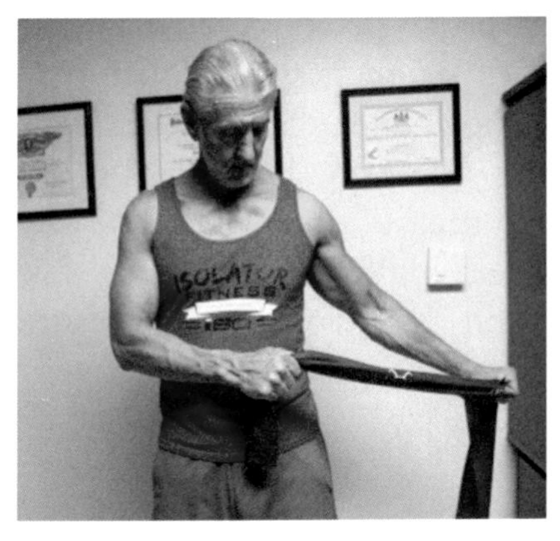
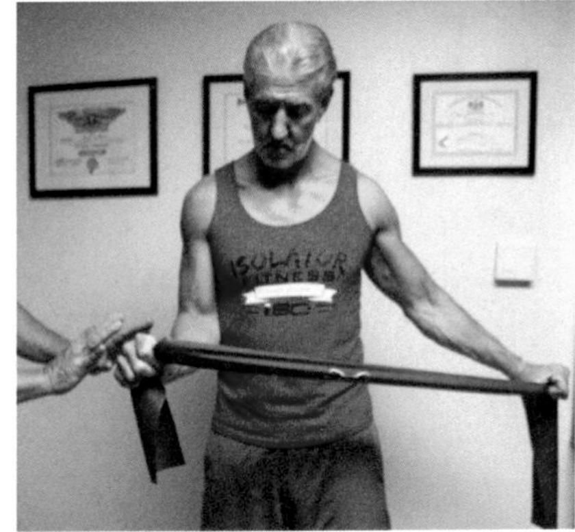

It's very important to work the rotator cuff in a short, specific range of motion. Make sure to look at the videos on my website, DrDeanWolf.com. If you have any doubt on how to train the shoulder, I'll show you several different ways to properly exercise this very important muscle group. It is paramount not to exercise the muscles that work in the opposite direction while trying to strengthen the cuff. Not to mention, you can generate more translation and pain when you exercise the wrong muscles.

Posture Deformity

A congenital translation problem in the shoulder is seen in people that have so-called "bad posture." This is a very common disorder and another leading cause of rotator cuff injuries in young athletes. Not to mention, it's not aesthetically pleasing. Having a nice posture gives a person less shoulder and upper back pain, making them look statuesque. "Bad posture" is one condition that can be successfully treated through scapulothoracic exercises. Scapulothoracic exercises are any exercises that pull the shoulders back. When doing these exercises, I try to feel my wing bones being pulled together. We have a couple of great videos on my website showing ways to get rid of poor posture, which will eliminate lower neck and upper back achiness, check them out at DrDeanWolf.com.

People that have posture issues typically have upper back and neck pain. I tell my patients to experiment with upper back and shoulder exercises. Some examples include changing hand positions or elevating or lowering the arm. Finding the one that isolates the "spot" or targeted area of achiness is the key. Shoulder retraction exercises help strengthen the muscles that pull the shoulder back. As shown on the following top picture, I have found rhomboid extension exercises are very effective in reducing posture issues. As well as any lat retraction exercises as shown on the bottom picture.

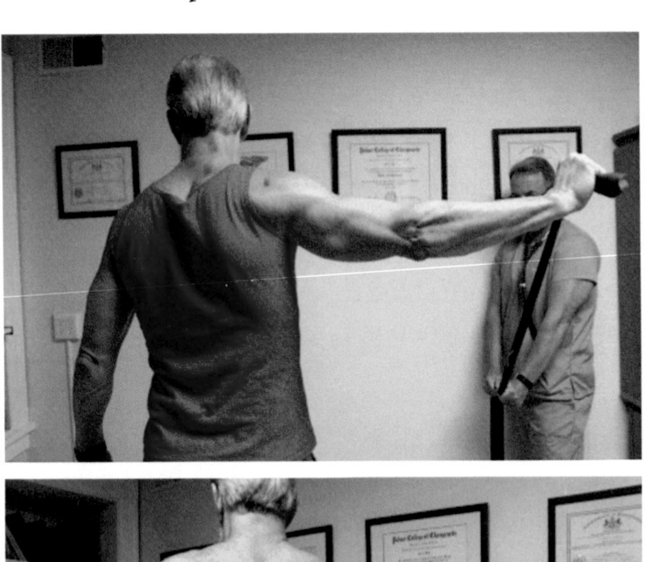

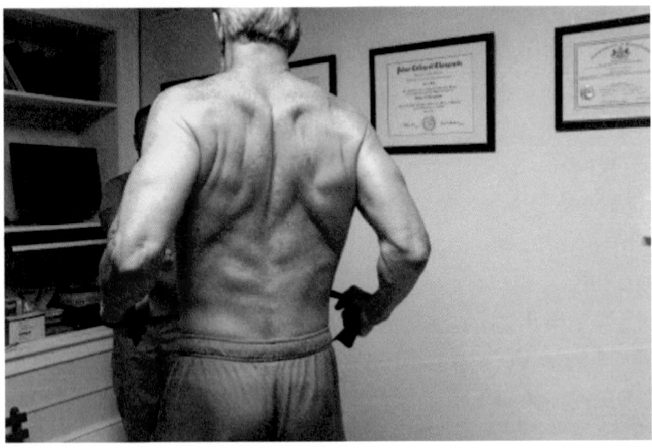

Knee

The next problematic joint is the knee. Let's review a few of the basic structures of the knee. There are four ligaments: *the anterior cruciate, the posterior cruciate,* and *the medial and lateral collateral ligaments*. We also have two pieces of cartilage: *namely, the medial and lateral meniscus*. There is a pretty big tendon in the front called the patellar tendon. Lastly, we have the kneecap, called the *patella*.

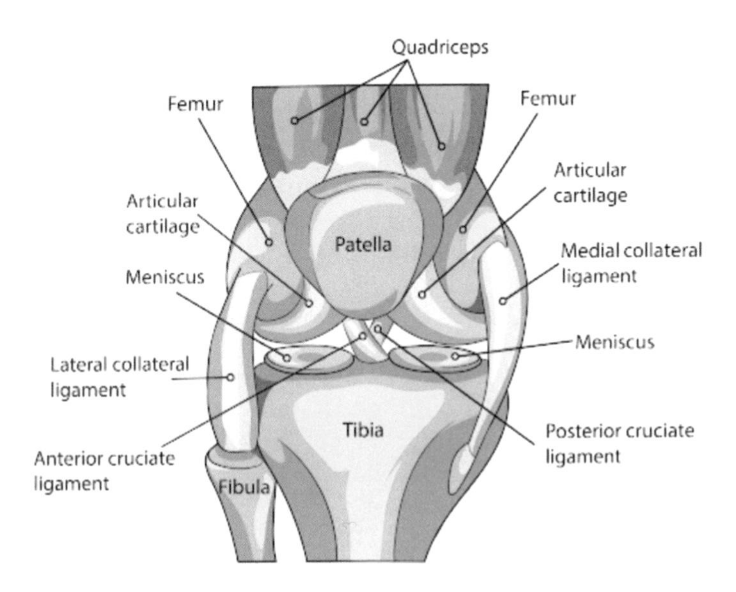

The most common translation deformity in the knee is anterior translation of the tibia due to hypermobility or injury to the anterior cruciate ligament (ACL). This is very common in athletes and ex-athletes. There are many knee injuries that are not due to translation issues. We will talk more of those injuries and how to treat them in Chapter 9. For now, let's discuss instability of the ACL. The anterior cruciate ligament is the primary stabilizer of the front of the knee. The hamstrings are the secondary stabilizers of the front of the knee and they help the ACL do its thing. So anytime we have ACL problems, the stronger the hamstrings are, the more likely we will be able to compensate for the loss of ACL stability.

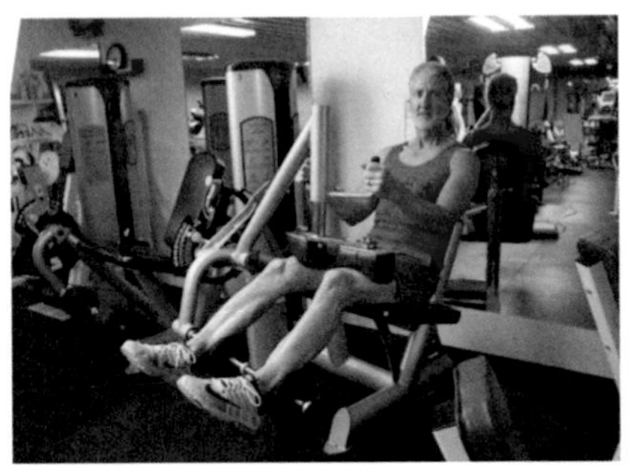

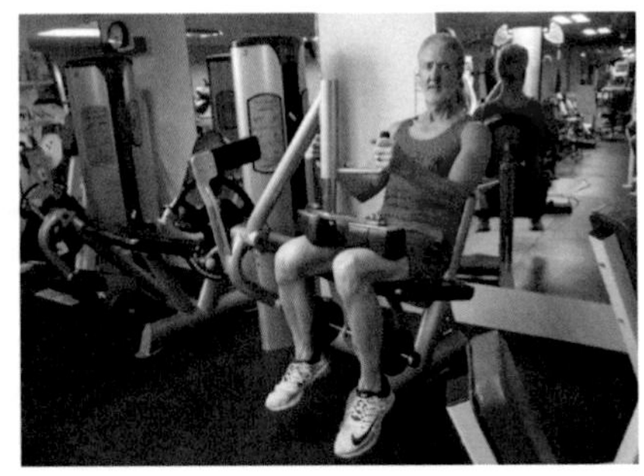

Interestingly, if there's mild ACL instability, the other structures can get injured. Because of the ACL translation, the hamstrings have to work harder to stabilize the knee. A person with ACL translation will be more prone to tendinitis issues and pulled hamstrings. Strengthening the hamstrings mitigates the instability caused by the weak ACL and usually gets the soreness out of the hamstring and its tendons. Additionally, working the quadriceps helps with the stability of the knee.

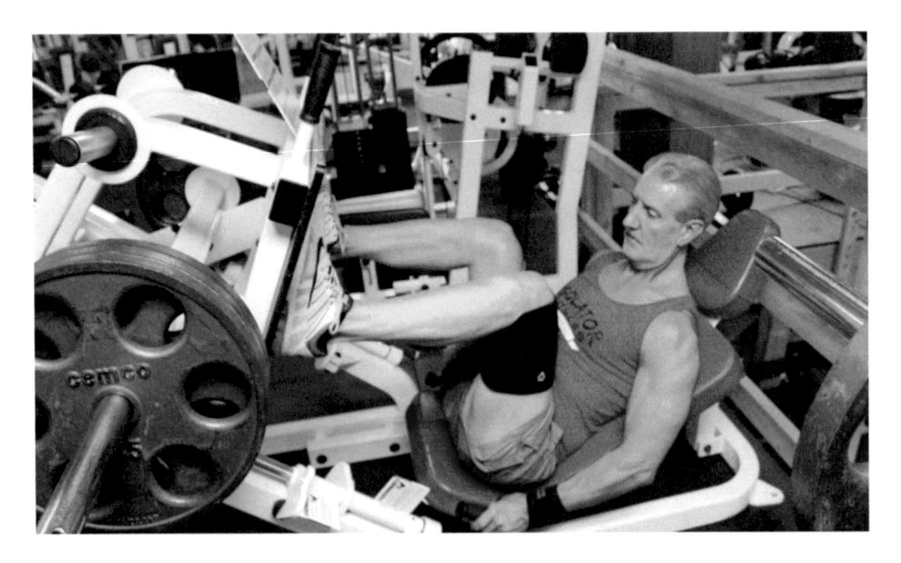

Since we have four ligaments, two pieces of cartilage and numerous muscular and tendinous attachments to the knee. It's important to have knees evaluated by a chiropractor or orthopedist to see if there are any injuries that could need surgical intervention. General strengthening of the quadriceps and hamstrings help a multitude of knee issues. We will get to more of these in Chapter 9.

Spine

The spine has two types of translation etiologies: degenerative disc disease and degenerative joint disease. Discs play such an important role in stabilization of the spine. Any dehydration of the disc between the vertebrae results in hypermobility. Translation deformity is a major cause of spine pain. It can be caused by disc degeneration or by degenerative joint changes to the joints in the facets. That's the case whether it's neck or low back pain. The vertebrae stack on top of one another like bricks on the wall of a building. When you bend forward, backward or side to side, these bricks shouldn't move or slip on top of one another. The diagram below shows how movement will affect a healthy spine.

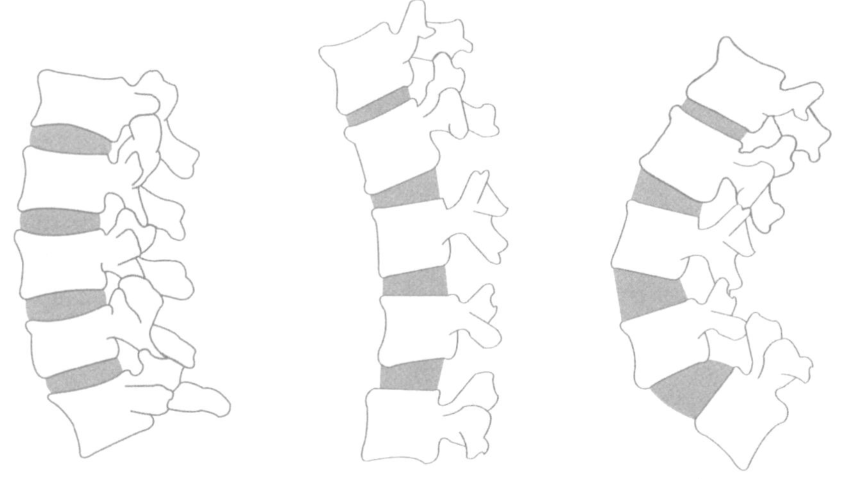

Neutral Position *Forward Movement* *Backward Movement*

The next diagram on the following page shows how these vertebrae slip over top one another (translation) resulting in pain. In the spine, translation can have neurologic consequences.

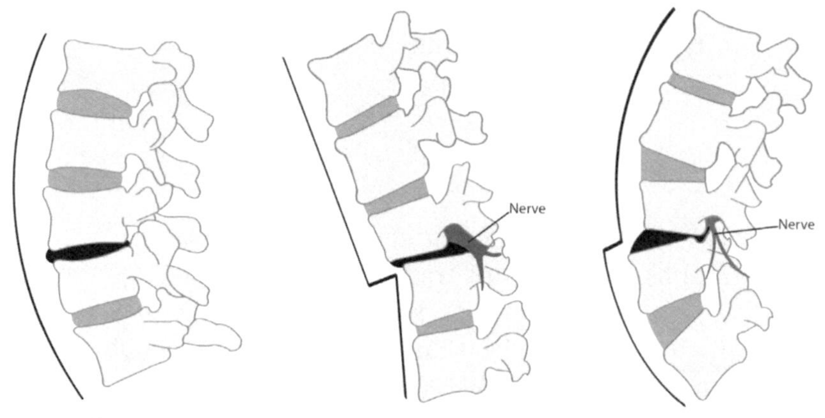

Neutral Position
No Translation

Forward Movement
w/ Resulting Translation

Backward Movement
w/ Resulting Translation

As this continual microtrauma occurs, the patient will start to experience inflammation in the facet joint or the disc, thus beginning the domino effect of a bad disc contributing to wear-and-tear on the facet joint, and a bad facet joint causing wear-and-tear on the disc. Both result in pain and perpetuating laxity.

When dealing with the knees and shoulders, we like to work the surrounding muscles to help strengthen the affected joint. The spine has more complex problems associated with it. The biggest problem with spinal instability and rehabilitation is that we do not want to exacerbate the root causes of the pain. So, putting a sore arthritic joint or a bad disc through a range of motion can be problematic in the spine. I found core exercises and cardiovascular training to be the most effective in the general strengthening of the muscles along the spine. If we strengthen our arms, legs, and core, the body's innate intelligence is going to maintain a degree of symmetry throughout our spinal muscles. In other words, the back and neck muscles will get stronger indirectly. In the next chapter section "O" we discuss the synergistic effect in more detail which will help you understand how to compensate for spinal instability problems. If you do core training and are working the abdominal muscles, it's imperative not to do full sit-ups if there is low back pain. They are recipes for a herniated disc. We will review proper abdominal exercises in Chapter 5.

CHAPTER FIVE

Weight Training. Let's Get Stronger!

There are an infinite number of ways to work out. For example, some people say the best way is through high repetitions and low weight. Others say low reps and high weight. In this chapter, I am going to show you how to get stronger. Then, I will show you some exercise techniques that will help minimize injury, tell you the facts and dispel myths, and show you how to strategically make the best use of your time in the gym.

A) Golden Rules

Let's introduce some time-tested golden rules when it comes to weight training. If you want to get rich, it's probably a good idea to ask someone who created their own wealth. The same is true for working out. I look to the professionals. I'm not talking about the college professors with PhDs in biochemistry who have never worked out and have a size 10 shirt collar. I'm talking about bodybuilders. Say what you want, these guys know how to do it. I'm not interested in getting 24" biceps or injecting anabolic steroids, but I am interested in getting stronger. I've spent time with former Mr. Olympia champions, logged countless hours in the gym, and read thousands of research papers and articles on building muscle mass. After all of that, I have come to the conclusion that there are four fundamental rules to building muscle after 40 or 50.

1) Eat Protein!
2) Put a muscle under tension!
3) Recover!
4) Recover!

1) Diet

Sounds pretty simple, right? Competitive bodybuilders say bodybuilding is 75% diet and 25% exercise. You are what you eat. We discussed earlier how protein is the material that builds things in our bodies – skin, organ tissue, everything. If you want to get stronger, you have to give your body the building blocks to make the tissue. Remember, spaghetti doesn't do anything to build muscle, just as motor oil doesn't make your car go faster. We went into detail the differences between carbohydrates and protein in Chapter 1. So, focus on the protein content of your foods. I found eating about 1 gram of protein per pound of body weight per day works great. Competitive bodybuilders eat much more. For our purposes, 1 gram per pound is a good rule of thumb. Not to mention, age and metabolism is a factor that 26 year-old bodybuilders don't worry about. Eat protein and get strong!

2) Time Under Tension

The second rule is to put the muscle under tension. Time under tension is what determines the amount of gains. The longer a muscle is under stress, the more damage occurs to it on a microscopic level. That's what we want. We need to beat them up so your body's innate intelligence says, "Let's rebuild those muscles stronger so they can better handle the stress placed on them the next time." Any time you lift weights and put the muscle under tension for an extended amount of time, you will build more muscle. That is why which training technique to use isn't as important as just plain exercising. You can exercise with long sets and a lot of quick repetitions or short sets with slow repetitions. The longer the muscle is under tension, the stronger it gets. In the long run, you will gain more muscle mass doing sets of 10 to 15 repetitions with lighter weights than doing 6 repetitions with heavier weights because of the longer amount of time under tension. Not to mention, you increase your likelihood for injury with heavier weight as you get older. Additionally, moving the weight slowly increases muscle mass more efficiently because of the overall time that the muscle has been under tension. Here again, the slower you go when you exercise a muscle, the less likely to incur injury as we get older.

3) Make Sure You Recover

I didn't stutter on Rules 3 and 4. Recovery is an extremely essential part of getting stronger. Lack of correct recovery time is the single biggest factor in the failure to make strength gains in our elder years. I remember reading a magazine article about a bodybuilder who had won the Mr. Olympia contest in his 40s. He stated that after all the years of training, he finally learned to recover. He learned that the longer his recovery period was between workouts, the better his gains. I have another example from my college days about how important recovery is for gains. My friends and I would work out in my basement doing bench presses and curls every Monday, Wednesday, and Friday. Then, we would go home for Christmas break for 2 weeks. Upon returning to college, we were amazed at the strength gains made during the layoff. We were working out the same muscle groups way too often. When we finally gave our muscles a break, we made larger strength gains.

Recovery is always very important, even at a young age, but it becomes even more important as we get older. The most common training flaw is getting back to the gym and tearing up the muscle fibers (myomeres) of the muscle before they've had enough time to repair. The following sentence might be the most important one in this book. After age 40, YOU SHOULD NEVER WORK OUT THE SAME MUSCLE GROUP MORE THAN 1 TIME A WEEK! You can be in the gym everyday, but work on different muscles each time.

B) Break Up Body Parts

Let's talk about the types of routines in the gym. I'll show you how I do it so you can then customize your own regimen based on your schedule. I break up my body into several parts for exercise. Optimally, I would like to get into the gym 5 days a week for training.

Monday: ARMS – bicep and tricep exercises

Tuesday: SHOULDERS – rotator cuff, deltoid and trapezius exercises

Wednesday: BACK – lats, rhomboids and scapulothoracic retractor exercises

Thursday: LEGS – calves, quads*, hamstring and glute exercises

Friday: UTILITY DAY – hip flexors, abs, internal and external hip rotation, chest* exercises

** I no longer perform some of these exercises due to my age. I will expand on this in Section J, Toxic Exercises.*

I call my fifth day a "utility day" because my goal is to get to the gym 5 days a week. Half of the time, I only make it 3 or 4 days. If your schedule is very dynamic and your ability to get to the gym varies, you should try to prioritize your workouts based on things to do because of injuries or genetic weaknesses. For example, if you have bad posture, I would make Day 1 "back exercise day." Or if you have knee issues, I would make "leg day" my number one priority. As a man, my favorite day is my "arms day." If I only make it to the gym 1 day a week, I'll do arm routines. My second priority is shoulders, which is why it's Day 2. Because I have translation deformity problems with my shoulders, I try to keep them strong to avoid injury. If I only get to the gym 3 times a week, my legs and utility exercises get skipped.

Now, if you only have 2 or 3 days to work out, you can combine muscle groups. For example, when you do back exercises, you work your biceps more than your triceps. So, back and biceps go together, as do chest and triceps. A three-day workout plan might look like this:

Monday: Chest and Triceps
Wednesday: Back and Biceps
Friday: Legs

C) Duration of Work Out

Many ask, "How long should I work out?" I like to keep my weight lifting routines to a flat 50 minutes. One of my good friends works out 90 minutes. I think that's too long. I'd rather get in and get out of there. Wearing my headphones, I tune out of the world for 50 minutes. I concentrate on time under tension. This 50 minute time frame must be kept focused and free from all distractions. I don't do a lot of talking when I'm working out. I want to hammer my muscles and get out of the gym.

D) Sets and Repetitions

Next, we need to figure out how many sets and reps we should do. Let's use my arm day for an example. I'll do 4 sets of 15 bicep repetitions for each individual exercise. Then I do 2 other sets of 15 reps, but these exercises will be different. In total, that's

12 sets of biceps and 12 sets of triceps with 15 reps each. Also, I like to alternate the sets. I'll do a bicep exercise, followed by a tricep exercise. This gives the muscles a little more recovery time between sets. My routine will take me 45-50 minutes. A typical day would be like this:

First 4 Sets of Bicep and Tricep routines:

First Set of Biceps	15 reps of curls with a curling bar, working the biceps
First Set of Triceps	15 reps of skull crushers, working the triceps
Second Set of Biceps	Second set of 15 reps with the curling bar
Second Set of Triceps	Second set of 15 reps of skull crushers
Third Set of Biceps	Third set of curls with curling bar
Third Set of Triceps	Third set of skull crushers
Fourth Set of Biceps	Fourth set of curls
Fourth Set of Triceps	Fourth set of skull crushers

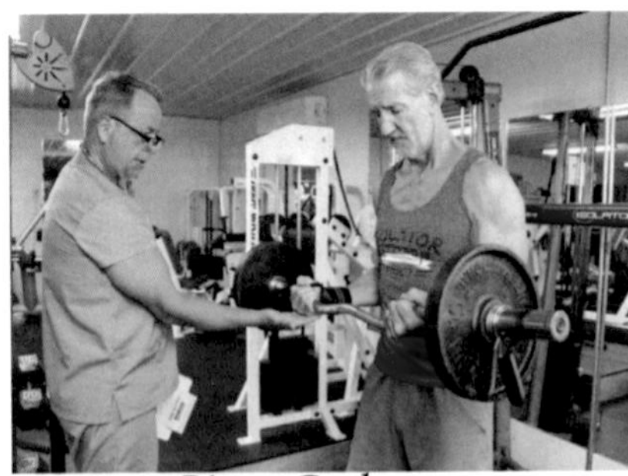

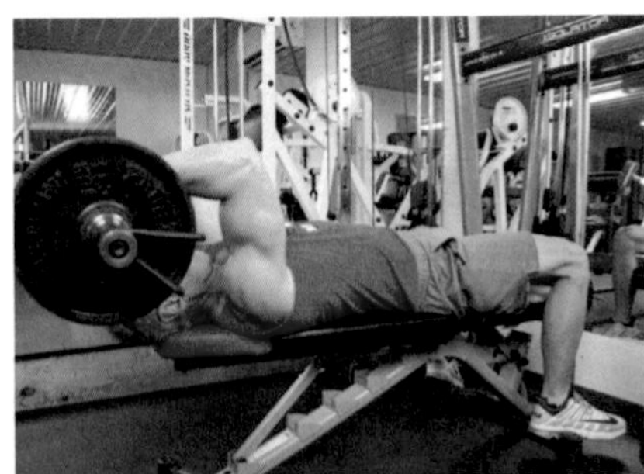

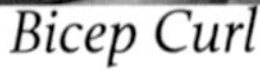

Bicep Curl

Tricep Skull Crusher

Then the fifth through the eighth sets of bicep and tricep routines:

Fifth Set of Biceps	First set of 15 reps of hammer curls
Fifth Set of Triceps	First set of 15 reps of kick backs
Sixth Set of Biceps	Second set of hammer curls
Sixth Set of Triceps	Second set of kick backs
Seventh Set of Biceps	Third set of hammer curls
Seventh Set of Triceps	Third set of kick backs
Eighth Set of Biceps	Fourth set of hammer curls
Eighth Set of Triceps	Fourth set of kick backs

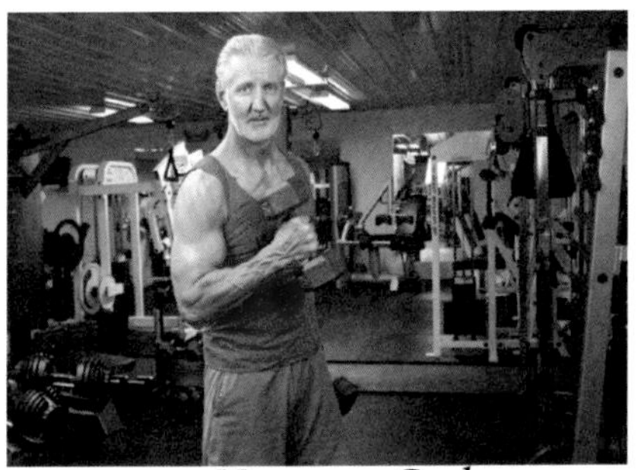
Hammer Curls

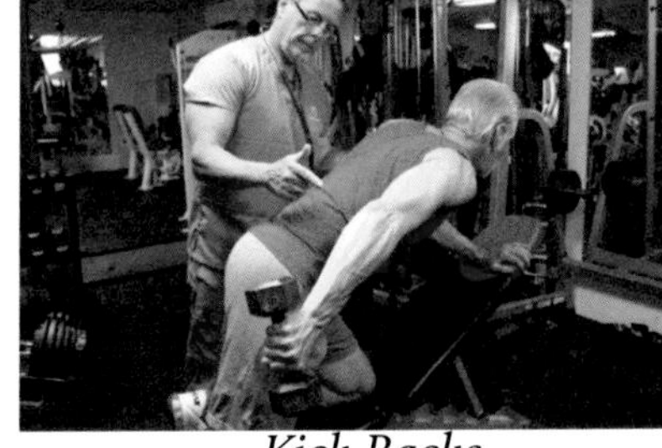
Kick Backs

Then, I'll switch to my third grouping of biceps and triceps exercises:

Ninth Set of Biceps	First set of cable curls, 15 reps
Ninth Set of Biceps	First set of cable presses, 15 reps
Tenth set of biceps	Second set of cable curls
Tenth set of triceps	Second set of cable presses
Elventh set of biceps	Third set of cable curls
Elventh set of triceps	Third set of cable presses
Twelfth set of biceps	Fourth set of cable curls
Twelfth set of triceps	Fourth set of cable presses

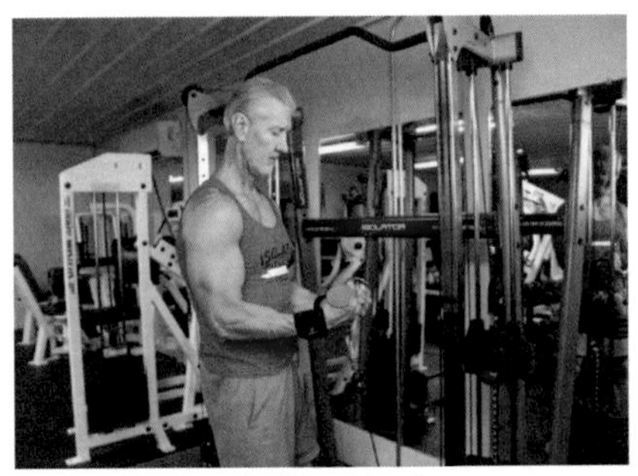

Cable Curls

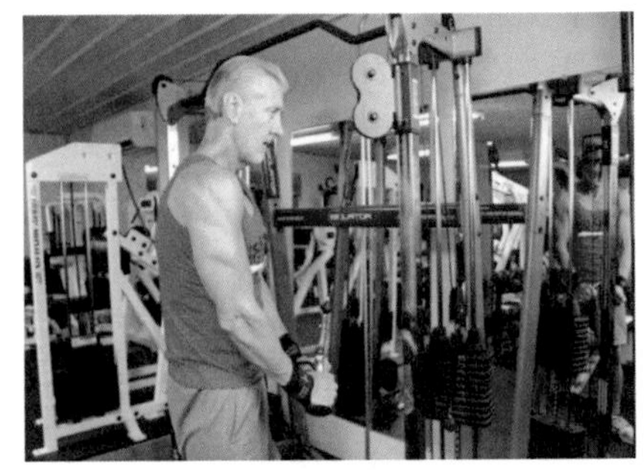

Cable Presses

There are several ways to do your sets. Supersets, agonist/antagonist training, pyramid training, and many others. (1) I like the pyramid method by far for the simple reason I can measure gains daily, not monthly. Here's how it works:

E) Pyramid Method

Let's say I do a tricep exercise. I'll start with a 30 lb dumbbell because I can easily handle the weight. I'll do a set of 15 reps. I'll do it nice and slow to warm up the muscles, but more importantly, I'll avoid injury because I am also warming up the tendons. My second set will be with 35 lbs. Not too hard to handle. A good load on the muscle and we're getting blood flowing into the tissues. My third set will be with 40 lbs. It's starting to get difficult now, yet I can handle it. This is when I will be sweating and breathing heavier. My fourth set will be with 45 lbs. In this hypothetical example, I would only be able to get this weight up about 6-7 times. The fact that I was unable to do the fourth set 15 times indicates that the weight I choose on the first set was about right. If I'm giving my body the right recovery, the next week that I perform this exercise, I should be able to do the 45 lb dumbbell 7-8 times. When you train properly, these are the gains you should see. In the first couple of months, you will see fast gains by adding at least an additional rep or two on the fourth set each time you workout. When your fourth set has reached 15 repetitions, you'll know you're ready to bump up your first set by one unit of weight - 5 lbs, in this case. When you start the same routine at 35 lbs on your first set, you will see that once you increase your weight increment, you will only be able to do 6-7 reps of 50 lbs on the last set. That's how easy it is. I love this technique because it covers all the bases. You get an adequate warm-up and you can chart gains. Seeing progressive gains keeps you motivated.

F) Muscle Confusion

Once you decide on a weekly routine, you should apply a few tricks that will help keep your gains coming. One of these tricks is called "muscle confusion." Our muscles get used to specific stresses placed on them. This slows down your gains. When working a particular muscle, we should occasionally change our routines to hit slightly different angles of the muscle. I found that I like to change routines every 3 months. As stated earlier, I'm doing 12 total tricep sets on my arm day. After 3 months, I'll find three different ways to do a tricep exercise. I might use the cable column, incorporate therabands, or even change my body position with free weights to achieve this.

Another form of muscle confusion is to change repetitions and weight. I do this at least once a year. If I did 15 repetitions with a 25 pound dumbbell, I'll change to doing 30 to 50 repetitions with a 15 lb dumbbell. This really gets my muscles burning. I'll use this method while training for my next 3-month cycle. Every year when I do this technique, I'm amazed at how sore I am the first few times. Our bodies clearly get used to the same routine. Switching it up every 3 months will help muscles make gains. If you have a translation problem with one of your joints, sometimes the pyramid technique might cause pain because of the heavier weight. In those instances, you might want to try lower weight with higher repetitions. With some exercises, I will do the pyramid method, but with other exercises, I'll go lightweight with a lot of repetitions. Let discomfort in the joint be your guide. You need to stress the muscle, not the joint. Time under tension is the most important thing. Even though you are working with less weight and more repetitions, the muscle is still under tension.

G) Chart Your Gains

When working out, it's a great idea to chart your routines. Write down how many reps and how many sets of each exercise you do. Keeping a log of what exercises you do is simple. By doing this, you can see your strengths and weaknesses. You can see how far you have come. You will find it exciting to look back through your old charts and see the gains made versus when you started. This keeps you motivated and focused. Also, I think it helps fight off that little devil inside all of us. You know, the one that tries to talk you into making deals to cut your workout short because you're tired, or persuades you to think that fourth set isn't necessary today. Simply charting all your routines helps to motivate and foster self-compliance.

H) Strength Versus Endurance

There's a lot of discussion regarding training for strength versus training for endurance. More repetitions performed with lighter weights yield benefits for endurance; fewer repetitions with heavier weights typically help you gain more strength. Regarding this principle, I'm convinced through my experience that the differences with weight training are minimal when compared to those of aerobic training – meaning there's an obvious difference between how marathon runners and sprinters train. I've trained using higher weight and less repetitions and found my mass gains are similar to less weight and higher reps. As we get older, it's better to train with lighter weights and higher reps. Once again, it reduces the chance of injury.

I) Use Short-Lever Techniques

In Chapter 4, I referred to translation deformity problems and their role in injury. As we age, the connective tissue in our bodies lose resilience. The matrix of the connective tissue loses water. This loss of fundamental fluid makes the tissue brittle. Unfortunately, we are stuck with this form of degeneration. Just as you can't restore the rubber of an old tire by placing it into a bucket of water, you can't expect to renew tissue by drinking water. Therefore, we need to train in such a way that will not create cracks in compromised tissue. Shorter ranges of motion in most exercises accomplish this nicely. Take curls, for example. When doing a curl, the first 40% of the motion puts a huge load on the tendon. Remember from Chapters 3 and 4, the tendon is the structure that connects the muscle to the bone. I see little benefit in putting the tendon under this load. This is the range of motion that creates tendinitis injuries and tendonosis problems. To decrease the likelihood of tendon injury, let's perform these motions in the last 60% of the range of motion. By shortening the lever of this exercise, we concentrate more on putting tension on the muscle instead of the tendon. You can see in the following picture that, at this point in the exercise, there is a lot of strain on the biceps tendon:

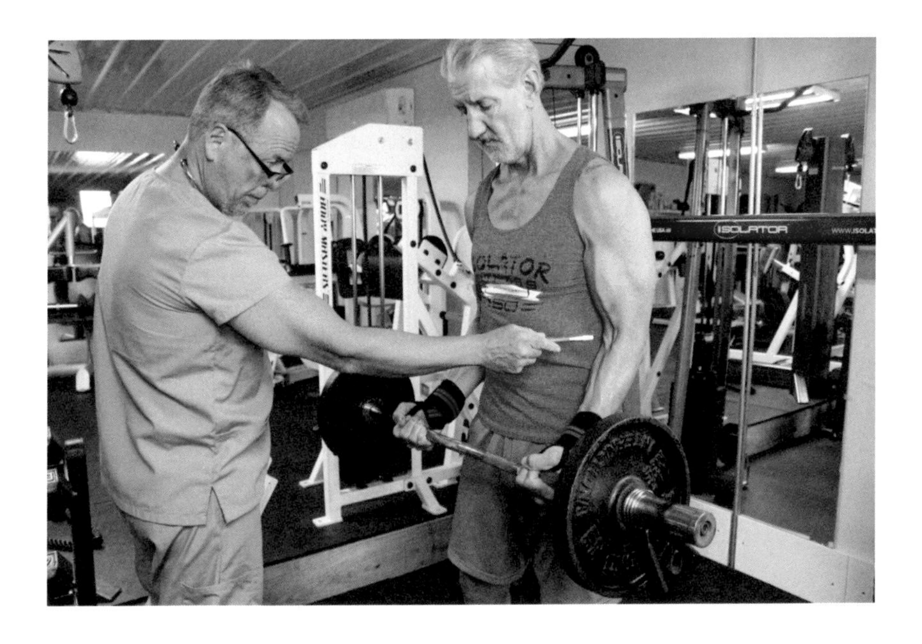

All you have to do is start the range of motion as you see in the following picture to eliminate excess strain on the connective tissue:

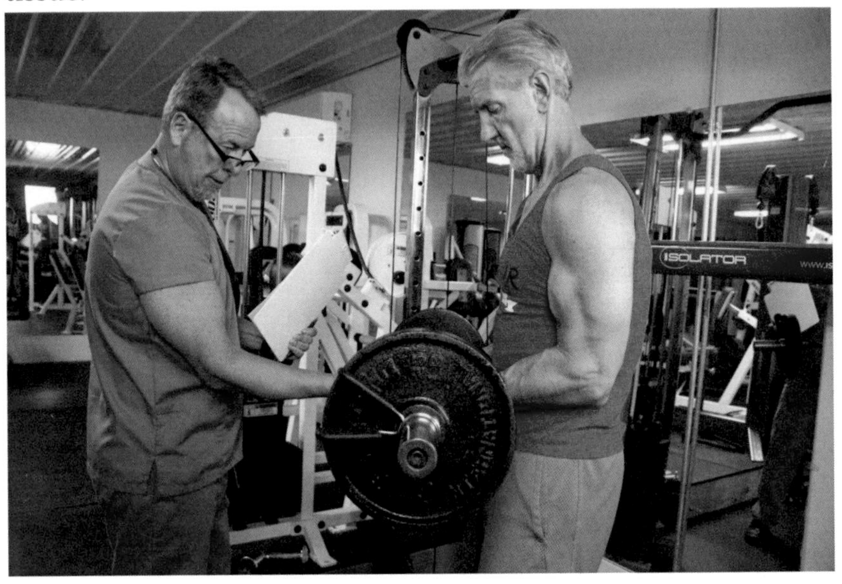

We can apply this principle to any exercise we perform at the gym. If you feel strain or unnatural tension on the tendon, shorten your lever on the tendon by exercising in the last 50-75% of the range of motion.

J) Avoid Toxic Exercises

There are several exercises that I call time bombs for injury: bench press, deadlifts, sit-ups, and squats. The oblique machine – in which a person sits and twists side-to-side – is a time bomb, too. I'm always tempted to put my chiropractic business cards next to this machine – it's a prescription for a herniated disc. After 50, if you do these exercises, you will get injured sooner or later.

In Section B of this chapter, you might have noticed two asterisks. Because of my age, I cannot do two of my favorite exercises anymore. I don't work my chest and I don't work my lateral quads. Chest exercises, including bench press, are a major reason I see patients in my office for shoulder injuries after age 40. I will address the mechanism of this in the Nuts and Bolts section of this chapter. (2) For the most part, we can exercise our chest in our 40s without too much of a problem. But once we hit the 50s, we are asking for trouble. I don't advise it for the simple reason it creates impingement in your shoulder, meaning the soft tissues get jammed together. I just think it's wise to avoid chest routines if you have any shoulder discomfort. That said, one of my best buddies is 56 and still does bench press without issue. Our bodies are wonderfully wired. If there's discomfort when exercising, don't do it. If you don't have pain, you generally have the green light. Here's one of the few ways I can do chest routines without creating impingement:

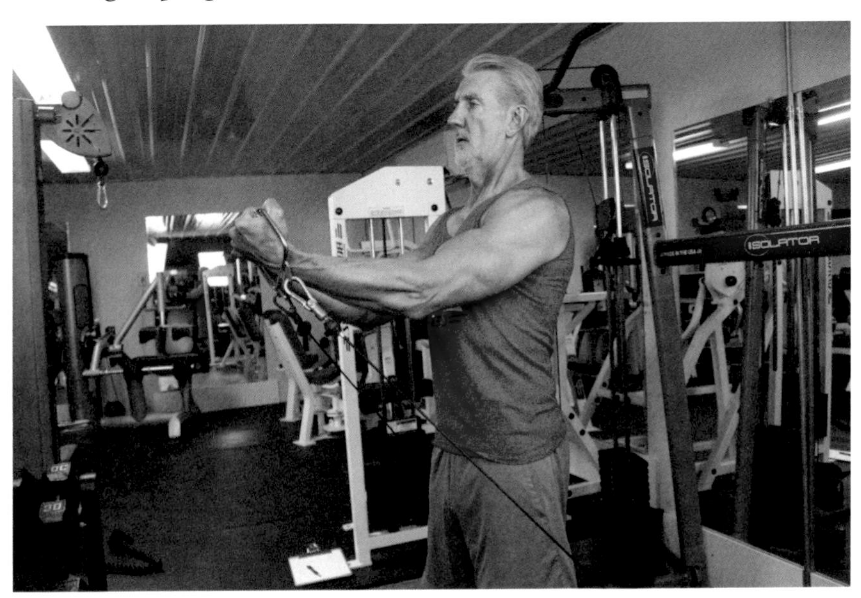

This next paragraph is going to raise eyebrows and generate controversy. When doing leg routines, I work the inner quad muscle called the vastus medialis. There are several mechanical problems that occur in the knee when the medial quad gets weak. I do this with leg extensions as shown below.

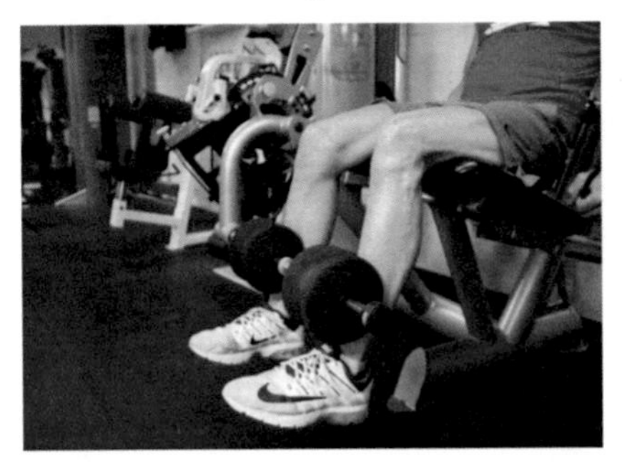

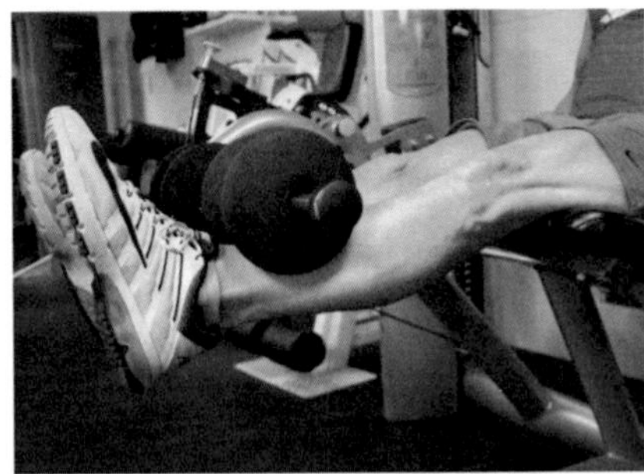

However, I don't work the other three quadriceps muscles. Here's why I don't work the other three quad muscles: I hate being so sore that I can barely walk for 3 or 4 days after doing those routines!!! I used to dread leg day. I'd think about my plans for the week to determine if I'd do my leg routine. If I knew I was playing golf over the weekend or going bowling with friends, I wouldn't do legs because my soreness would affect my performance. Then it occurred to me, "Why do I even do legs? I use them every day. I use them going up steps and down steps, getting out of a chair or car, and a tremendous amount during cardio training." We use our legs all the time.

Think about this next statement. In 30 years of practice, I've never had someone come into my office with a problem that was a manifestation of a weak middle or lateral quadriceps – namely, the vastus intermedius, vastus lateralis or rectus femoris, the three quads in question here. However, there are many problems that occur because of weakness in the medial quadriceps – the vastus medialis. This muscle is the innermost front thigh muscle. It's important to keep this one strong. We will address several disorders that occur from a weak medial quad muscle in Chapter 9 in the knee section of this book.

Furthermore, there is one last problem with quads. They are the strongest muscles in the body. When exercising them, you are able to use hundreds of pounds of weight. When we get in our 40s and 50s, the cartilage in your knee and hips lose water. The tissue becomes more fragile. Putting a huge amount of weight-bearing stress into these cartilage compartments is the cause of many injuries. Muscles can regrow and regenerate; cartilage cannot. I have first-hand experience with this. I tore my labrum in my hip while doing heavy lunges with dumbbells when I was 51. Meniscal tears in the knee are common with leg press and squat exercises. Additionally, squats cause progression of degenerative disc and joint changes in the lumbar spine. I have treated hundreds of patients who are weight lifters in their late-20s and early-30s for disc herniations. These athletes just won't stop doing squats and deadlifts. The following MRI is a 26 year-old bodybuilder with multiple compression fractures and severe disc degeneration from doing deadlifts and squats with hundreds of pounds of weight. It's pure physics, their muscles are strong enough to lift more weight than their frame can handle.

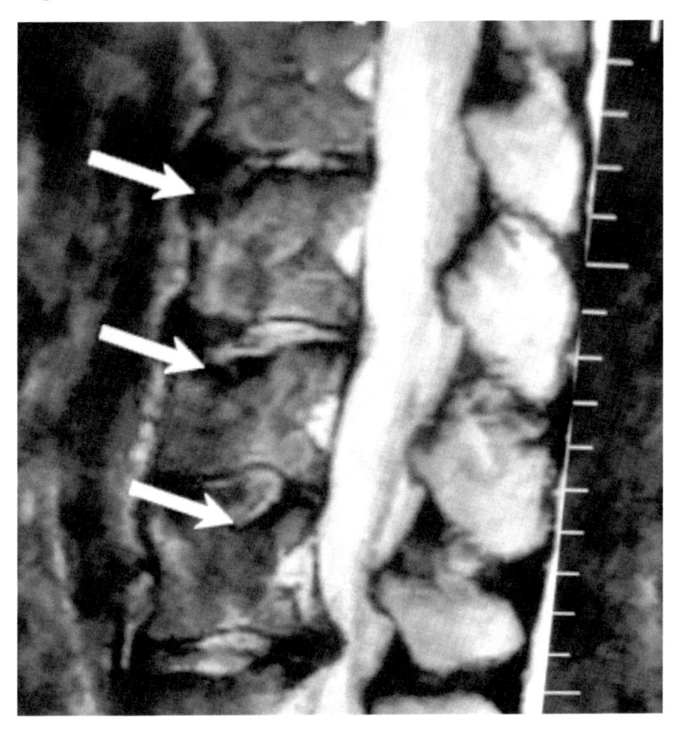

Because these movements are power exercises, I completely understand why they are fun and rewarding. Squats and deadlifts are the two power exercises that just shouldn't be performed if you're in or above the 40 or 50 age range. Once again, let your innate intelligence be the guide. Our goal is to get fit and look great. We don't want to do things that put us on the perpetual injured reserve list.

Sit-ups are another exercise that we should not do. There are a lot of great ways to exercise the abs without causing injury to the back. Working the rectus abdominis, your 6-pack, doesn't flatten the stomach anyway. To the contrary, working your abs can make your stomach bigger. Cardiovascular exercise is more useful if you would like to shred the excess weight that hides sculpted abdominal muscles. Even some bodybuilders lose sight of this one. If you want to flatten your stomach, I suggest you stress the internal obliques. This is a great exercise for toning your stomach. Get into the sit-up position, lift your rear end off the ground, and then try to do a sit-up. As long as your pelvis is not touching the ground, you can exercise your abs without creating any stress into the low back.

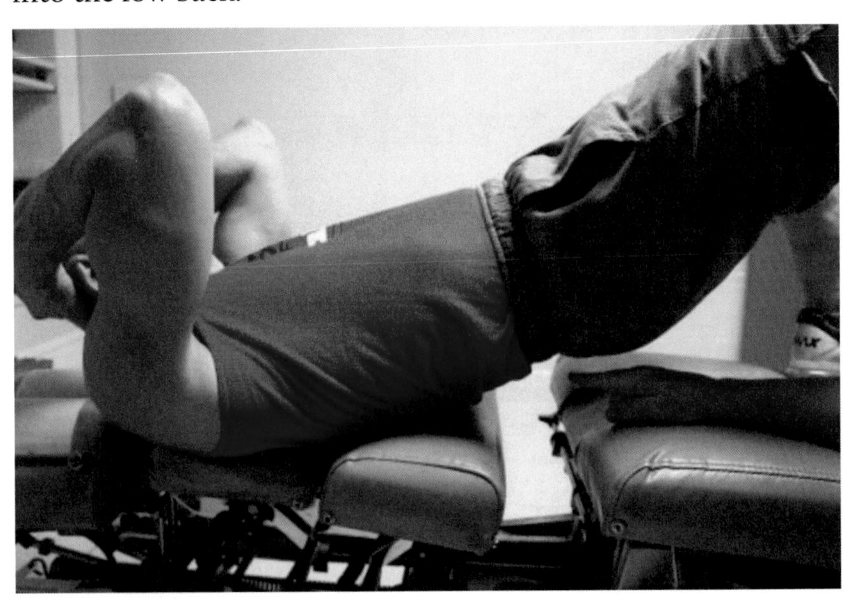

Biomechanically, the pelvis and sacrum function as the fulcrum point when doing sit-ups. As you lift your torso off the ground, a tremendous amount of shear occurs into the bottom disc of your low back.

If you have low back pain, chances are you have a degenerative disc or two. The sit-up motion causes shear into the disc and the resultant translation of the bones. This shear creates microscopic cracks in the outside (annulus) of the disc. Anyone that's been diagnosed with degenerative disc disease of the lumbar spine will tell you their back hurts when they do sit-ups. If you don't have degenerative disc disease and you keep doing sit-ups after age 50, you will get low back pain eventually. The first half of the full sit-up motion is poison to your low back. When working your abdominal area, this is the perfect time to practice the principle of shortening the long lever like we mentioned in section I. When I do abdominal routines, I get on a decline board and put it on its highest notch. Then I exercise in the last 50% of the range of motion.

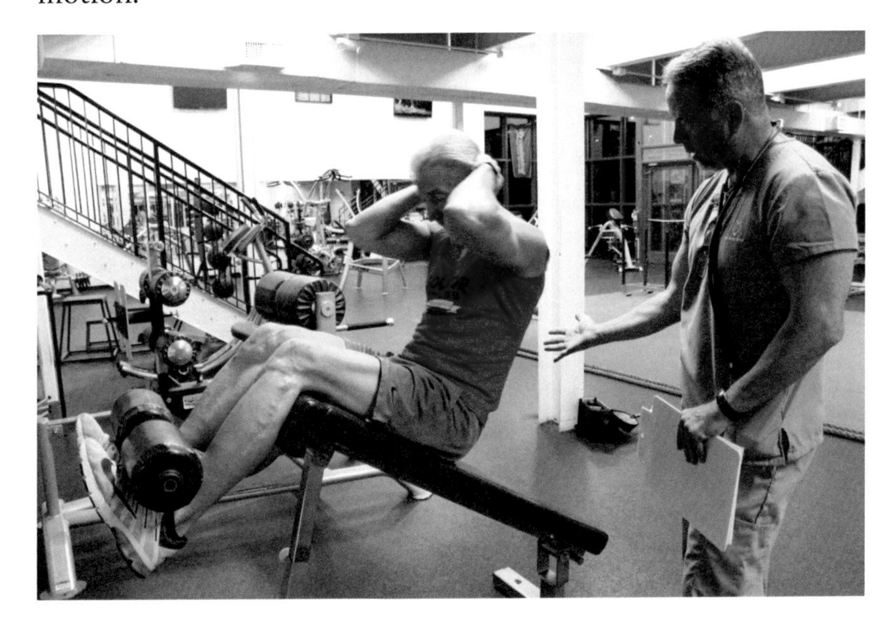

Some exercises can be toxic while other routines can work the same muscle group with no mechanical wear and tear to the joints. A perfect example of this is calf exercises. Most gyms have a machine that exercises the calf muscles. But some of these pieces of equipment can cause injury. A perfect example is the machine with the shoulder pads that a person raises by standing on their toes.

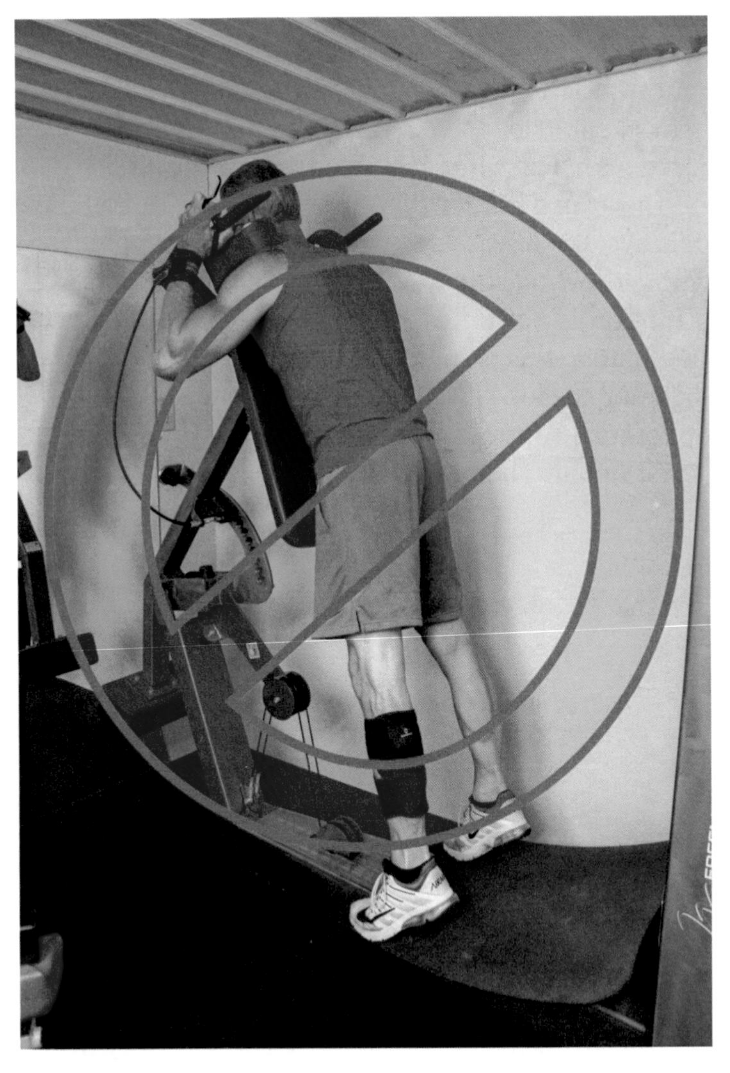

While this machine clearly works your calf muscles, you are compressing your spine with hundreds of pounds of weight in an effort to work your lower legs. Never compress the spine when exercising. This machine clearly advances degenerative disc disease after age 50. A better way of doing the same exercise is to use a leg press machine and do toe raises. This eliminates spinal compression; or, find a machine like this one:

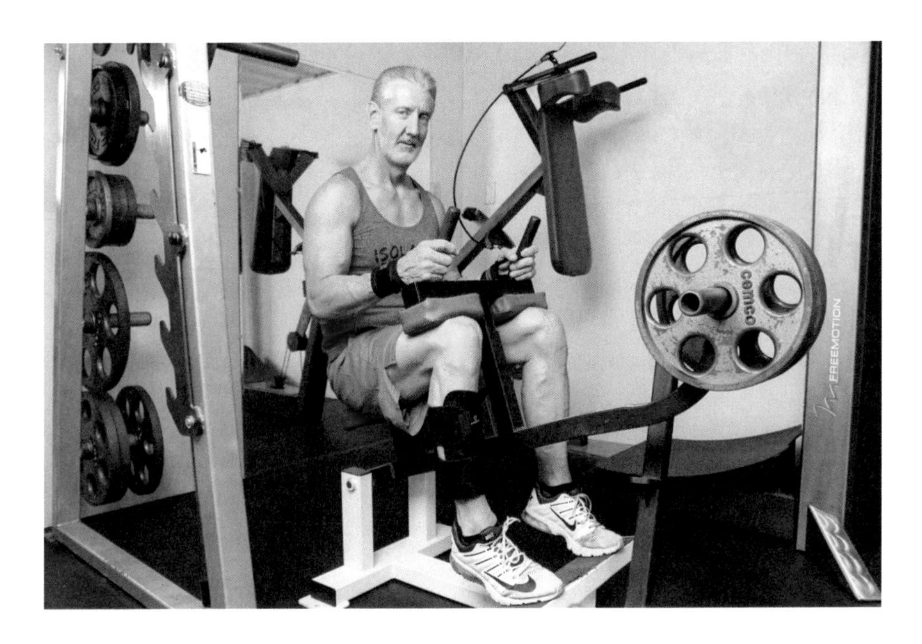

K) Warm Up and Warm Down

I think it's a great idea to get on the treadmill or elliptical trainer and warm up for 5 minutes before lifting weights. After the warm up, I weight train for 45-50 minutes, then do 30 minutes of cardio to finish. I love doing this for several reasons. When increasing your heart rate, thereby speeding up your metabolic processes, you enhance regeneration and repair. If your goal is to build muscles and get ripped, be careful not to do cardio longer than 30 minutes. After 30 minutes of aerobic activity, your body can break down muscle to make energy. (3) This does not help your cause. My goal is to look good and have great cardio endurance. Balance is the key. Personally, I don't want to have the physique of a marathon runner or that of a muscle-bound bodybuilder. My overall goal is a healthy balance of both. We will address cardio training in the next chapter.

L) Use Wight Lifting Tools

I use a few tools to help avoid injury when training. My favorite: the ISOGRIPPS™ (**isogripps.com**) made by Isolator Fitness. This product is one of the most awesome tools for the gym – you must have one of these!

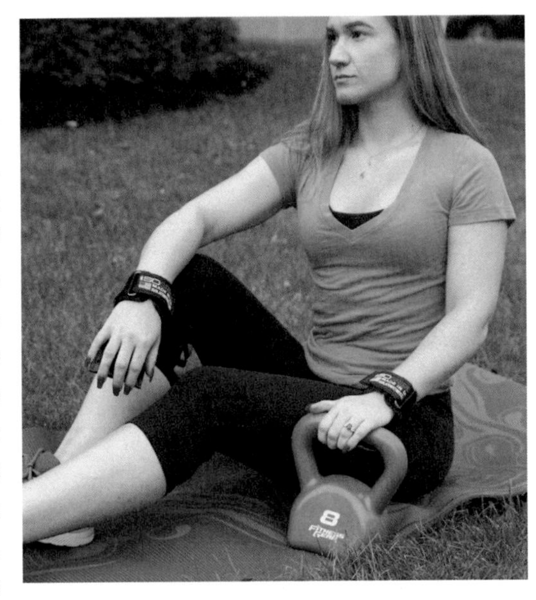

This gripping tool helps me handle heavy dumbbells for shoulder and back exercises that otherwise I couldn't perform because of hand strength. They are simple to use, and more importantly, can help avert wrist injury. The ISOGRIPPS™ are great for women, too. Because women generally have less hand strength, the ISOGRIPPS™ help them handle weight with less strain on the wrist.

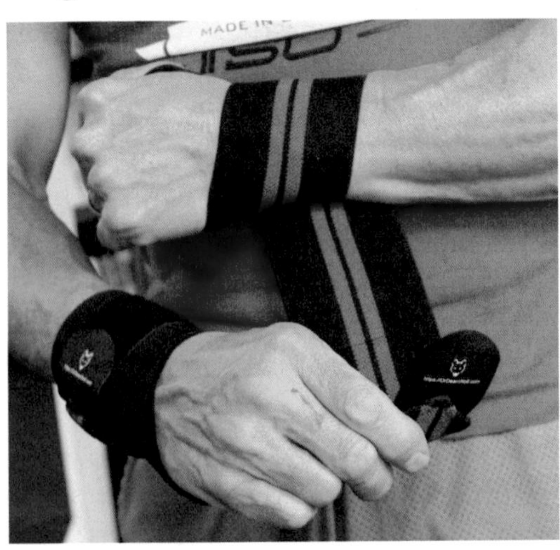

I like athletic wrist wraps when working out. This helps avoid wrist injury (**wolfwristwrap.com**).

Another helpful apparatus is called the Isolator. (**isolatorfitness.com**) This tool enables someone who has a hand injury to do any upper body exercises. While suffering from a bad case of tennis elbow, I threw a baseball to my son, causing injury to my rotator cuff. When trying to rehab my shoulder, I found I had a lot of pain in my elbow while doing my rotator cuff exercises. I tried the Isolator and was able to complete all my routines without any pain. This equipment can be used to help anyone who is an amputee or has a serious elbow, hand, or wrist injury work out.

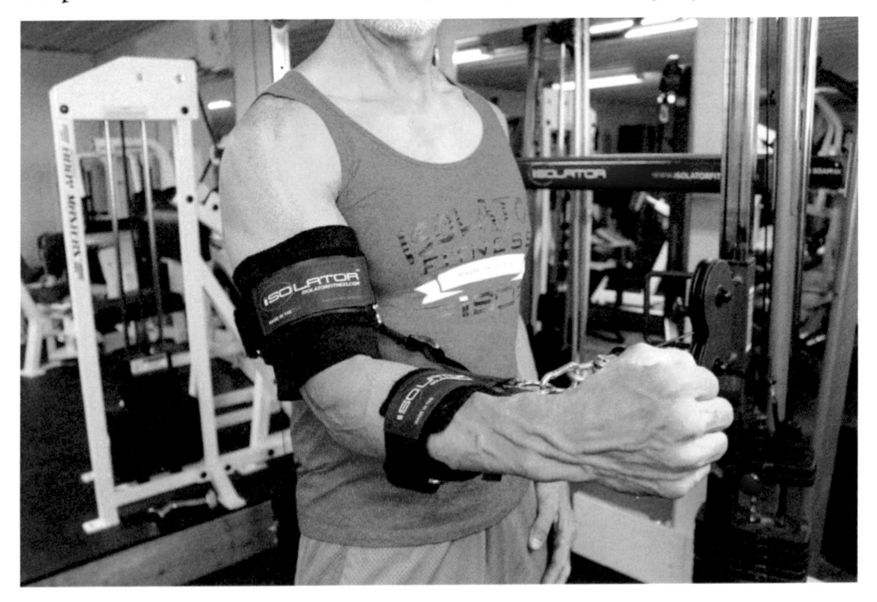

M) Use Supplements

The reason you see so many sports supplements out there is because they work. When I work out, I would feel naked without taking my protein and my aminos. Here's what I do. Right before I work out, I make a customized pre-workout drink. What's in it? I start with a scoop of nitric oxide (**wolfnitricshock.com**) and 20 grams of whey protein. Then, I add a tablespoon of type II collagen, 5 grams of creatine monohydrate (**wolfcreatine.com**), 5 grams of leucine and 5 grams of glutamine. I finish by mixing these ingredients in a blender to an easily drinkable consistency – it's so simple to do! While I'm at it, I mix up my post-workout drink. I add a liquid that naturally contains some sugar, like orange juice or milk, to a mix of 20 grams of protein and 5 grams each of creatine, leucine, and glutamine. The addition of something with sugar creates a spike in insulin, one of the strongest growth hormones. (4) Do not be intimidated by this process. I made a video showing how to do it. It's quick, easy, and tastes delicious. Just go to **DrDeanWolf.com**.

N) Genetic Predisposition

Our bodies have a set genetic makeup. We are predisposed to look a certain way. There are three body types: ectomorph, mesomorph, and endomorph. Body type can affect how you respond to diet and training. The ectomorph is a hardgainer, meaning this person has problems putting on muscle mass. His body looks skinny with a frail looking frame and usually a high metabolism. The mesomorph has a nice "V" shape body that most men desire to have. They are naturally strong and gain muscle mass the easiest. The mesomorph has a genetic advantage with training. Lastly, the endomorph has sort of the opposite physique of the mesomorph and most commonly has a stocky build and gains weight easily.

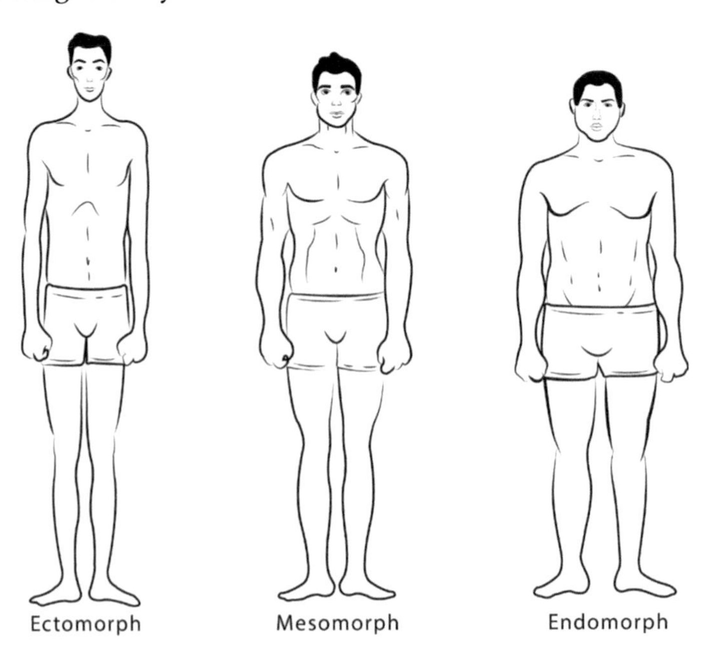

An ectomorph body type cannot look like a mesomorph, regardless of the amount of exercise. Muscle can be built on the ectomorph by going to the gym, thereby improving the body's physical presentation. I'm an endomorph. When I put on weight, it goes to my legs and stomach. When I train, my cardio reduces the body fat at undesirable areas and the weight lifting increases my upper body size, getting me closer to the desired mesomorph shape. By training properly, no matter your body type, you can improve your overall appearance.

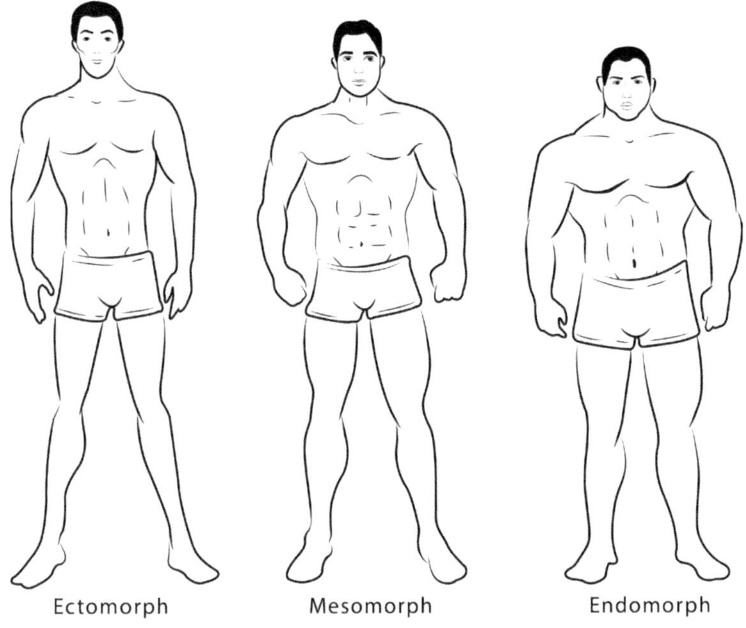

O) The Synergistic Effect

Lastly, when it comes to training, here's something to think about. There's a biological principle I've coined the "synergistic effect." I've heard it called other names, like "mirroring." Bodybuilders have known for years when they hit the point where they can't get their arms any bigger, they would concentrate hard on their legs. The old adage was "put an inch on your legs, and you'll put an inch on your arms." Chiropractors, orthopedic surgeons, and physical therapists alike notice working collateral and antagonistic body parts can have a therapeutic benefit to an injured area. We can use this physiologic principle of our own unique symmetry to our benefit. So if you have a body part or an area that you can't exercise because of structural injuries, work everything around them. I'll use myself as an example. I have severe bilateral translation deformity in both my shoulders. Chapter 4 was all about my loose shoulders. When I do a bench press, my shoulders hurt because of a translation affect. Almost every chest routine causes me discomfort. To counteract that, I work my shoulders to increase the muscle strength in that area. I especially work the rotator cuff. Then, I work my back, abs, and everything but my chest. Using conventional thinking, you would think I'd have nice arms, shoulders and a flat sunken chest. Interestingly, I've been told my chest is my best feature. While doing other routines, my chest muscles are being used to help stabilize my frame. For instance, if I'm doing dumbbell lat pulls on a bench, the contralateral pectoral muscles are firing to help stabilize my structure. This indirect way of putting the muscle under tension is another way our bodies maintain symmetry.

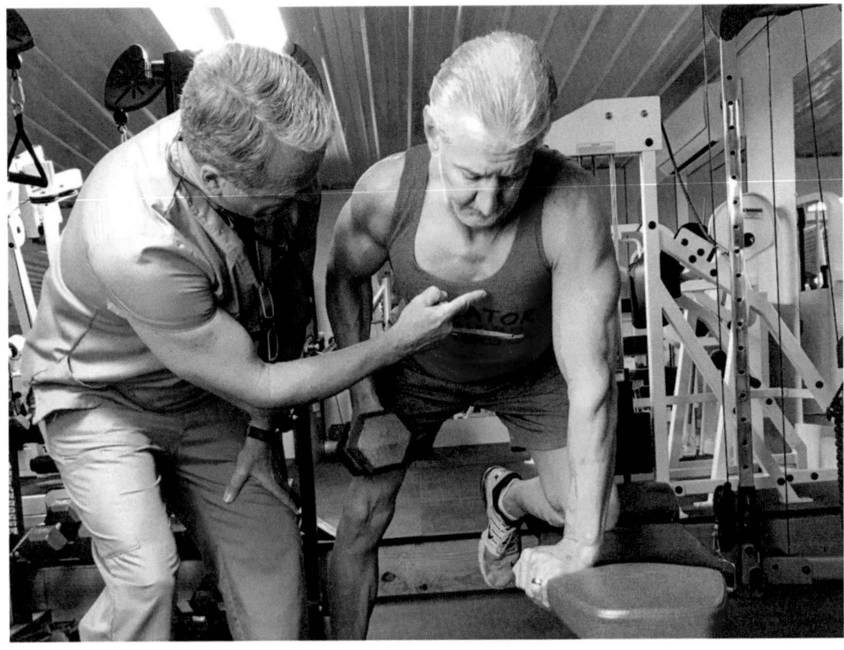

In conclusion, If you have a problem area, just work everything else around it. You'll see a collateral benefit to your trouble spots as your body maintains its own genetic makeup.

Nuts and Bolts

(1) Super sets are a good way of getting a great work out in less time because you move from one exercise to another quickly without rest. I also like to do high repetition sets. I love working agonist and antagonist muscles with this type of routine, meaning alternating opposing muscle groups, with 30-second rest periods. This saves time in the gym and I get a killer workout. An example would be doing a set of biceps, followed by doing a set of triceps. Additionally, I find an aerobic benefit when using this technique.

Calisthenics training is a great way to train if you don't go to the gym and do not have any weight lifting equipment at home. This would include push-ups, pull-ups, dips, and the like. Convenience and availability are strong points here. The problem I find with this type of training is boredom and the consequential lack of compliance.

Circuit training is another popular method. The person doing this type of routine goes from station to station to use different exercise machines, ultimately working all muscle groups several times a week. I'm not a fan. The only benefit in my mind is the resulting caloric burn from general activity. Some even say there is some aerobic benefit, but I believe any actual aerobic benefit is minimal. The biggest downside is reduced recovery. If you like to train using machines, try and work different muscle groups each time. We should only work a muscle group once a week.

(2) The shoulder joint presents a lot of biomechanical challenges when you want to do chest routines. Once your arms elevate to 70° or 80°, some impingement a rotator cuff tendon (supraspinatus tendon) occurs. Most chest routines involve the shoulder being abducted. As seen in the diagram on the following page, during abduction the acromion process of the scapula can jab right into the tendon. There are several different types of formations of this bone. If the acromion process is physically longer, it's more likely to compromise the shoulder tendons during abduction.

Impingement Syndrome

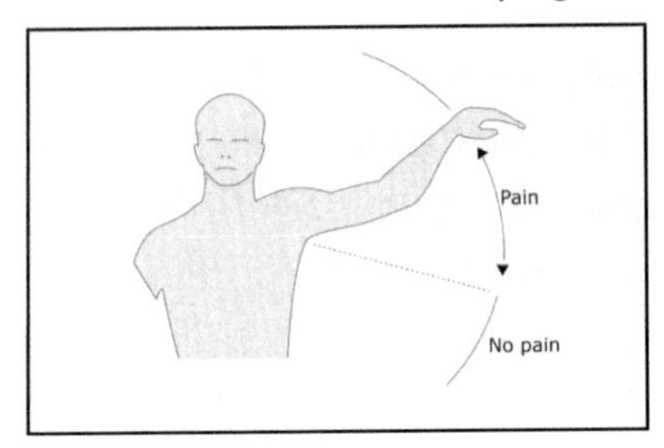

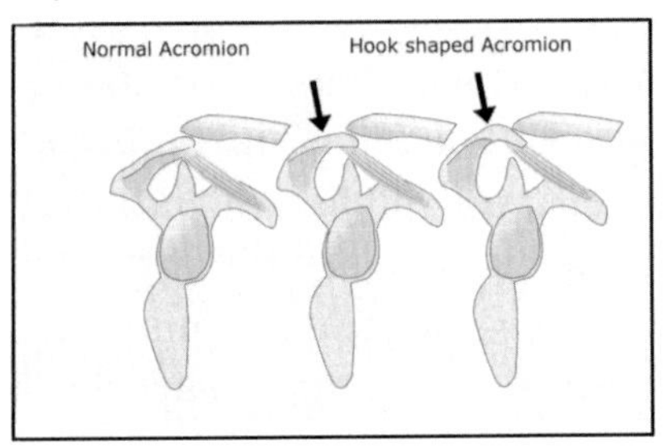

Additionally, this same problem occurs if there is a telescopic force put into the shoulder, such as the move performed during a bench press. The other mechanical issue with the shoulder as we age is joint translation. The joint capsule plays a role in the stability of the shoulder. When capsule laxity is present, the rotator cuff has to take up the slack. The four small muscles that make up the rotator cuff have a tall order when dealing with injuries associated with throwing. The rotator cuff decelerates the arm when throwing an object. It takes a lot of newtons of force to throw a baseball, and 3 times as much force to stop your arm. That's why baseball players and athletes alike commonly injure the rotator cuff. The strong muscles involved in throwing the ball rarely get hurt. I will expand on this topic in Chapter 9.

(3) Glycogen is a form of sugar that is stored in the body for energy. It is readily available to be turned into sugar for energy during exercise. The liver and muscles hold about 400 grams of glycogen. When the body loses enough sugar and energy-converted fat, it turns to the muscles to get some sugar. Gluconeogenesis is a metabolic process whereby sugar is formed by non-carbohydrate resources. When the body needs to replenish sugar, it will break down muscle tissue and convert it. This is a defense mechanism the body uses to maintain a constant sugar level needed for energy. This occurs when a person is in starvation mode from fasting or exercising for too long. When trying to build muscle mass, we want to be careful to not do anything that promotes

gluconeogenesis. This is exactly what happens to marathon runners. Their bodies use all the sugar reserves and are forced to tear down muscle to make more energy. Conversely, Olympic sprinters have very muscular physiques. The short quick burst exercise doesn't deplete glycogen stores. I have found a good rule of thumb: when it comes to aerobic training, do not go over 30 minutes. If your goal is to get lean, then 30-plus minutes of cardiovascular exercise will get this done. But if you want to build muscle mass, keep the cardio to 30 minutes or less.

(4) We know that insulin is the chemical that reduces blood sugar levels in our body. Additionally, it is a super powerful growth hormone. We can use this to our advantage. After working out, I like to mix something with sugar into my protein shake. This can be milk or fruit juice, depending on your palate. A lot of textbooks talk about the magical 30 to 60 minute window of time for optimal protein uptake. In essence, we are tricking our bodies to make some growth hormone right after we work out.

CHAPTER SIX

Aerobic Excercise

The Fountain of Youth

Aerobic activity is one of the best ways we can achieve the calorie deficit we are looking for when trying to lose weight. I call aerobic exercise "the fountain of youth" because I'm not sure if there is one thing we can do dietarily or actively that can have as many collateral health benefits. In this chapter, we will discuss how to exercise aerobically, how long to exercise, how hard to exercise, different types of aerobics, and ways to manage aerobic activity to achieve desired health benefits.

A) What is Aerobic Exercise?

Aerobic exercise means moderate to intense physical training that promotes a more efficient heart rate and use of oxygen when accommodating elevated biological activity. The result is an overall improved bodily condition. Basically, activity that makes you sweat and breathe vigorously results in a stronger heart, stronger arteries, and increased lung capacity. "Cardiovascular training" and "aerobic training" are synonyms that can be used interchangeably. Any activity that increases your heart rate can be considered aerobic. At what point does increased heart rate activity have a true positive biological effect on overall conditioning? I think the answer is any activity. So if you're in poor cardiac or vascular physical health and want to turn that around, any activity is a start. The important thing is to start! We will discuss ways to measure heart strength gains shortly.

B) Get a Physical

Because cardiovascular exercise puts an increased demand on the heart, it is important to get a physical examination to assess that it is safe to stress the heart muscle. At the least, you should have a doctor listen to your chest and do basic blood pressure readings to see if there is any reason to go to the next level of testing. Simply listening to your heart can identify mechanical abnormalities such as valvular problems. Blood pressure testing is about the easiest way to evaluate your overall vascular constitution. The best thing to do is to get a stress test. The nice thing about doing any preliminary evaluation is that you can get a baseline as to what your physical health is like, and then do the same tests later to see how aerobic training has had a dramatic effect on your overall health.

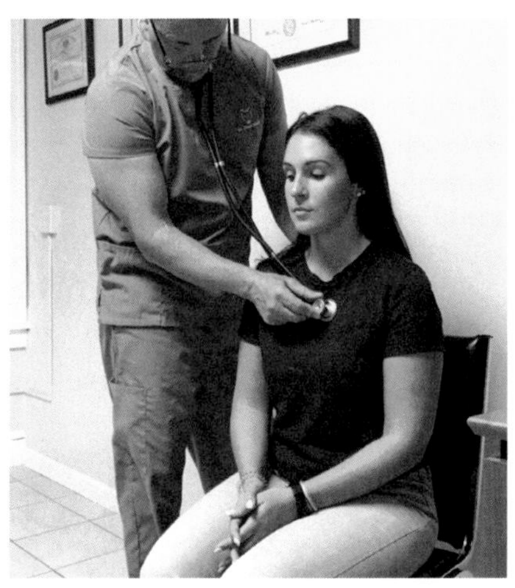

C) The Heart

First, let's talk about some physiologic basics. Heart rate is the amount of times a heart beats in a minute. Of course, resting heart rate is the amount of times in a minute that your heart beats at rest. This is a great indicator of overall vascular integrity itself. The reason being is because your body has a certain biological demand every minute. A certain amount of oxygen needs to flow through your system every minute to keep you alive. Not to mention, oxygen-fueled chemical exchanges occur in your body to control temperature, digestion, and a myriad of other activities. The average person has a resting heart rate of 72 beats per minute. So, it takes 72 beats of a heart to maintain the body's biological state in a minute of time during rest. If your resting heart rate is 80 beats per minute at rest, then we know your heart muscle is weaker than the guy whose heart beats 72 times per minute. Because the same amount of demand is there, a weak heart has to pump 80 times to accomplish what a healthy heart takes 72 to do. Conversely, if your resting heart rate is 60, we know that your heart is very strong because it accomplishes the same work in only 60 beats. (1)

D) What is Your Blood Pressure?

Next, there's blood pressure. Blood pressure is the measurement of the pressure of the circulation of blood on the walls of the blood vessels of your body. The two pressure readings are systolic and diastolic. Systolic pressure is the pressure on the walls of the major arteries when the heart pumps blood. Diastolic pressure is the pressure on the walls of the major arteries when the heart is at rest. These measurements are based on how much pressure it takes to raise elemental mercury a said amount of millimeters against gravity. A healthy blood pressure reading is 120/70. Typically, high blood pressure readings are defined when systolic pressure is over 140 and diastolic pressure is over 90. High blood pressure is often referred to as the silent killer because many people have high blood pressure with no outward symptoms. On the other hand, low blood pressure typically manifests itself in the form of fatigue.

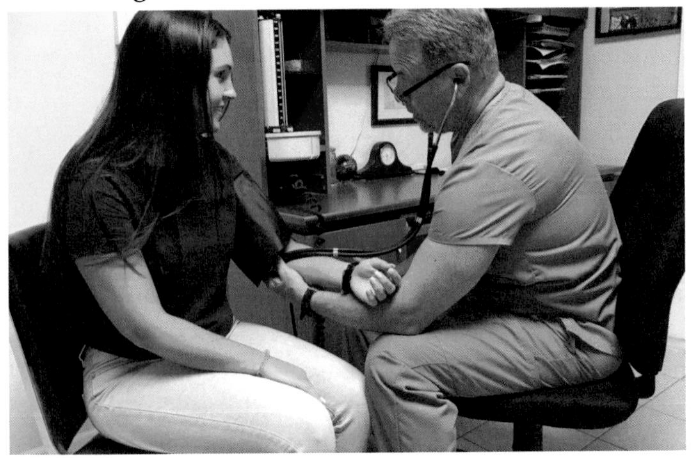

E) High Blood Pressure

There are several common causes of high blood pressure. Instead of putting this in the Nuts and Bolts section of this chapter, I'm going to try to tackle this one right now. I think it's good to understand the mechanism of how blood circulates through our body.

Basically, the anatomy of the vascular system consists of a pump and a bunch of pipes. The pump is the heart. There are two kinds of pipes. First, there are arteries. Arteries are responsible for carrying blood away from the heart. Second, there are veins. Veins are the structures that return blood to the heart. The major difference with these two types of pipes is that arteries have muscles in them and veins do not. When dissecting a body, you can differentiate the arteries from the veins by their volume, not their color. An artery looks cylindrical with body to it. The vein looks collapsed and flaccid with no cylindrical form. Now, here's the cool part. It's sort of incorrect to suggest that the heart pumps blood through our body. In reality, the heart pumps blood into a few major arteries. These arteries then contract and squeeze blood throughout our entire system. That is why you can feel a palpable beat when you put your finger on someone to get their pulse – and that is why your entire body doesn't pulsate every time your heart beats. This produces a very smooth laminar flow and is an awesome system.

Think of it like this. The job of the heart is to push blood into a few pipes. These pipes expand, and then smoothly contract. The amount of pressure it takes to push the blood into the arteries and get them to expand is "the blood pressure." So, what happens with high blood pressure? If blood pressure is high, it means that the heart has to contract harder to get the artery to expand and receive the blood. Here's the problem with making the heart work harder. When an increase in demand takes place, a muscle has to get bigger. It's nice when our biceps get bigger, but not our heart. The reason is because the heart is packed into a tight chest cavity.

There is very little room for it to expand. Unfortunately, this means it grows inward. This is a slow, progressive, and potentially fatal condition. Trying to breathe with an enlarged heart is like laying on your back and trying to breathe with someone sitting on your stomach. Hearts are built for endurance like a marathon runner's legs. We want our heart silhouette on a chest X-ray to be nice and small.

What could cause high blood pressure? Well, it could be because the arteries developed arteriosclerosis (thickening and hardening that occurs as we age). If the wall of the artery is hardened, it is difficult for the heart to push blood with enough force into the vessel to get it to expand. Another cause of hypertension (high blood pressure) is atherosclerosis, which is when a bunch of junk is stuck to the walls of the artery. Plaque makes the lumen (the opening of the artery) smaller, allowing less blood to get through. Another common cause of high blood pressure is increased blood plasma volume. If there is a lot more water flowing through the pipes, it takes more "pressure" to push everything through. Anyone that has an expandable garden hose can witness this phenomenon – the more water you turn on, the harder the hose gets. This expansion of volume can be caused by too much salt in our diet. For those with high blood pressure, in most cases just reducing our salt intake each day to under 2,300 mg can easily lower blood pressure by 10-20 points in a couple of weeks. The problem with continually having excess water in our pipes is if the "garden hose" is always full, the pipes harden over time. That's what arteriosclerosis is all about. We will explain the mechanism of salt on blood pressure in the Nuts and Bolts. (2)

F) Aerobic Benefit

Now that we are finished with Cardiology 101, let's talk about how to get started exercising aerobically. As I mentioned earlier, any activity that increases your heart rate is good. The benefits of activity need no explanation. However, at what point does the amount of activity increase the actual strength of the heart? This is defined as aerobic benefit. When in poor cardiovascular health, a little activity will have benefits. Experts agree that, for most of us, true cardiovascular strengthening occurs at about the 8- to 12-minute mark of aerobic training. The important thing is to exercise in the correct range. The chart below has the universally accepted ranges for heartbeat frequency. The chart shows the age and maximum heart rate for your age. It's good to exercise in the 80% range.

Age	80% Target Heart Rate	100% Maximum Heart Rate
20	160	200
30	152	190
40	144	180
50	136	170
60	128	160
70	120	150

G) Frequency and Duration

I am a firm believer in doing cardio for 15-30 minutes, all the while maintaining a heart rate at about 80% of your maximum capacity. This is where I love using my fitness tracker band or any other heart monitoring device. I find using these devices help keep track of your heart rate and expended calories quite nicely. In a short period of time, you will get to the point where you know what your heart rate is by how heavy you are breathing. If you stay in the 80% range, you'll find yourself breathing firmly and your body generating a good bit of perspiration. Going past the 80% range can cause danger. Remember, the idea is to train and get stronger – not destroy and get weaker. As discussed in the Nuts and Bolts from the last chapter, it's good to keep your cardio down to no more than 30 minutes if you're trying to build muscle. However, if your goal is to be lean, 60 minutes will do it.

The optimal number of days of aerobic training is 4-5 a week, I recommend a minimum of 3. Cardiac muscle is different from skeletal muscle. (3) The muscle fibers of the heart don't fatigue like that of skeletal muscle. So, we are able to work the heart muscle more often than our biceps. If I'm on a mission to lean out quickly, I might do cardio 6 days a week. I always take 1 day off. But of those 6 days, I might only do 3 days of what I call more intense training. Even with the heart muscle, we want some degree of recovery.

H) Aerobic Confusion

Another great way to increase your cardiovascular fitness is to do interval training. Interval training simply changes your pace throughout your routine. For 2-4 minutes, you might go at a moderate rate, then begin decelerating to a slow rate. After a few minutes, increase to an aggressive rate, then repeat the cycle. You'll find most treadmills, elliptical trainers, and stair steppers have a setting for different rates. This serves as an aerobic form of cardiac muscle confusion. When you are stuck on a plateau and finding it hard to make gains, this is a great jump starter. You will make quicker cardiovascular improvements with interval training as opposed to staying at the same pace.

I) Low Impact

I think the important thing when exercising aerobically is to keep the impact to a minimum. I'm not a big fan of running. For those that have good genetics and no knee or hip issues, the impact won't have much of a detrimental effect. But for most of us, the constant micro trauma from running will take its toll on the cartilage structures. Swimming is probably the least load bearing on the joints. Biking is great, too, and I find spin classes to be a lot of fun. My personal favorite is the elliptical trainer and a stair stepper.

J) Chart Your Workouts

My fitness tracker band charts my resting heart rate by day and weeks. It's amazing how fast you can improve your heart strength. When I start a 12-week cycle of eating super clean and exercise, I can, on average, lower my heart rate by 1 beat a week. I'll go from 70 beats per minute to the upper 50s in 12 weeks every time. On the other hand, when leading a deleterious lifestyle while on vacation, my resting heart rate can go up 1 beat in a day. This is another advantage to having a fitness tracker. It's useful to consistently monitor your physical conditioning for the simple fact that it gives you a little subconscious kick in the butt if you're getting too far off track with your lifestyle.

K) Fight Boredom

One of the advantages of running is that it is not boring. Being outside is nice because there's always something to look at. Boredom is the kryptonite of cardio. Finding a way to keep your cardio sessions interesting is no small task. Personally, I put on my noise-suppressing headphones and jam to my favorite music. Having a TV handy is another useful tool. I like to exercise in a public gym atmosphere because people-watching helps pass the time. Additionally, changing up your cardio routines helps fight boredom too. Some days, I'll do 15 minutes on the elliptical and 15 minutes on the stair stepper instead of all 30 minutes on the same machine.

L) Health Benefit

The benefits of aerobic training are innumerable. As your cardiovascular conditioning improves, your body becomes better equipped to handle oxygen transport from an increase in blood volume and lung capacity. This increase in volume has other effects, such as increased endurance with weight training, thereby mutually improving your ability to build muscle. Additionally, your athletic performance improves. Your tennis serve will be hotter; your tee ball will go longer. At the end of your matches, fatigue does not play the same role in decreasing performance. Then there are the obvious benefits of increased heart health, weight loss, and lowered blood pressure. Weight loss and aerobic conditioning help with other health issues as well. Many can get off diabetes medication by simply dropping a few pounds by eating right and getting some exercise. As we get stronger, we have less susceptibility to injury.

Another major health benefit to aerobic training is an increase in HDL levels in your blood. HDL is commonly referred to as good cholesterol. These high-density lipoproteins play a role in cleaning out your arteries and reversing cardiovascular disease. Chapter 1, Nuts and Bolts: Number 1 discusses the benefits of HDLs.

Studies have shown that cardiovascular exercise helps improve your cognitive skills. Sleep improvements have been directly related to aerobic training. Not to mention, cardio creates an increase in endorphin and enkephalin production. These are the body's neurotransmitters that are responsible for a sense of well being. One of the best ways to fight depression is to work out aerobically. Another mental health benefit cardio gives us is a vehicle to get tension and psychological stress out of our body. Maybe the greatest silent benefit to aerobic conditioning is that sexual health is greatly improved. Since you're not running out of steam, your physical performance improves and, as a direct result, you build confidence - and your mate is happy, too. All these things help to make you more productive in your daily activities with increased energy and vitality.

M) Exercising at Night

Some studies have shown that exercising at various times of day can yield different results. I'm not a big fan of studies. You'll notice I don't quote studies in this book. After 30 years as a practicing chiropractor and seeing so many theories debunked, I find myself to be cynical regarding the scientific community. Their results are typically agenda driven. They can produce a study to show "with great scientific certainty" two completely different outcomes with the same data. Another frustration I have with the scientific community is that their interpretations of the data are, more than not, tied to political motivations. Even with that said, I have found several good studies that reinforce the fact that exercising at night is more useful for increasing your metabolic rate versus exercising in the morning. The higher your metabolic rate, the more weight you lose. This increased rate is responsible for more muscle gains; however, exercising in the morning or afternoon is still much better than not exercising at all.

I have personally experienced increased weight loss from exercising at night versus exercising in the morning. Here's the catch: I am less compliant with exercise at night. While there is a slight increase in benefit, I have found it's not worth the risk of skipping the gym because I'm tired after a long day. So, I usually exercise in the morning or afternoon.

When you go on a diet without any aerobic or anaerobic training, most of what you lose is muscle. This also reinforces our understanding as to why people that go on crash diets without exercise look weak and frail – they are losing too much muscle. Aerobic activity helps prevent muscle loss and increases fat loss. Not to mention, any increase in muscle weight increases your basal metabolic rate. There is no better way to be healthy and feel great than doing cardiovascular exercise. (4)

Nuts and Bolts

(1) Stroke Volume. The left ventricle of your heart pumps blood into the aorta, which is the largest artery in the body. About two-thirds of the blood in the ventricle gets pumped out on any one contraction. So, stroke volume is the amount of blood pumped out of the heart with each cycle. This can be measured with an ultrasound test. Aerobic training increases heart muscle strength, thereby increasing the stroke volume. Since more blood is getting pumped out with each beat, your heart can beat fewer times to get the same job done.

(2) The mechanism that salt has on raising blood pressure is a function of osmosis. When two water bodies are divided by a semipermeable membrane, water will move through the membrane from the side with a higher concentration of particles to the lower side. Bodies of water like to have the same concentrations of particles. Simply put, it's a law of nature that particles in a solution like to be in even concentrations. So, here's what happens in our bodies. When we eat salt, it passes out of our intestines and into the bloodstream. Now, there are more particles per unit volume of space in the bloodstream versus the interstitial spaces outside of the artery. Then, osmosis kicks in and water moves into the artery to balance the concentrations of particles inside and outside. We have a problem now. More water in the artery means more pressure on the walls of the arteries. Consequently, the heart has to work harder to push everything through the pipes. All of this puts extra strain on the heart and arteries. This is probably the easiest health hazard to avoid. By simply keeping your salt intake to a minimum, you ensure less blood pressure and less stress on the heart.

(3) Cardiac muscle and skeletal muscle are completely different. Cardiac muscle is built for endurance and skeletal muscle is built for performance. When skeletal muscle is put under stress, it gets larger to compensate for the increased demand on the tissue. This can't happen with cardiac muscle because there is no space

to enlarge. The heart has a much larger blood supply than skeletal muscles to help reduce fatigue. Additionally, the heart muscle cells have many more mitochondria than their skeletal counterparts. Mitochondria is a power plant of a cell.

(4) Cardiovascular exercise can increase your metabolic rate. Here's how this works. As discussed in Chapter 1, the basal metabolic rate is the rate of energy your body uses to maintain itself. After a night of sleep, we feel a bit tired at first. As we wake up and move around throughout the day, our body processes kick into overdrive: the heart rate is up, thoughts occur, and food is digested along with a ton of other body regulations. As night falls, we start to become tired. This is when our metabolic rate is the lowest.

The following charts demonstrate the changes in metabolic activity throughout the day: the slow increase when we get up in the morning; the peak energy output levels in mid-afternoon; and finally, the slow decrease afterward. For purposes of explanation, we will say that this chart represents a 2,000 calorie a day metabolism with no exercise.

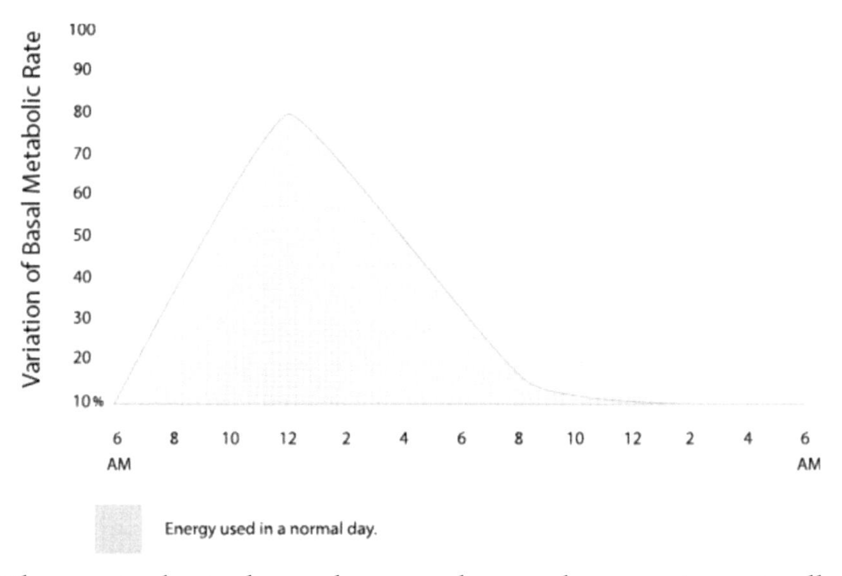

The next chart shows how cardiovascular exercise actually increases your metabolic rate. Exercise was performed in the morning. The shaded area represents a net gain of energy expended.

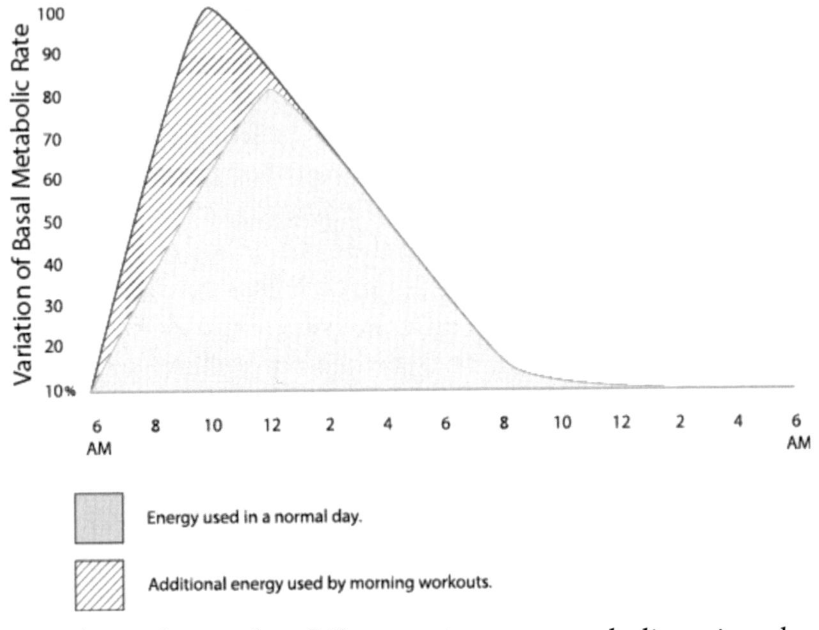

This chart shows the difference in net metabolic gain when exercising in the evening hours.

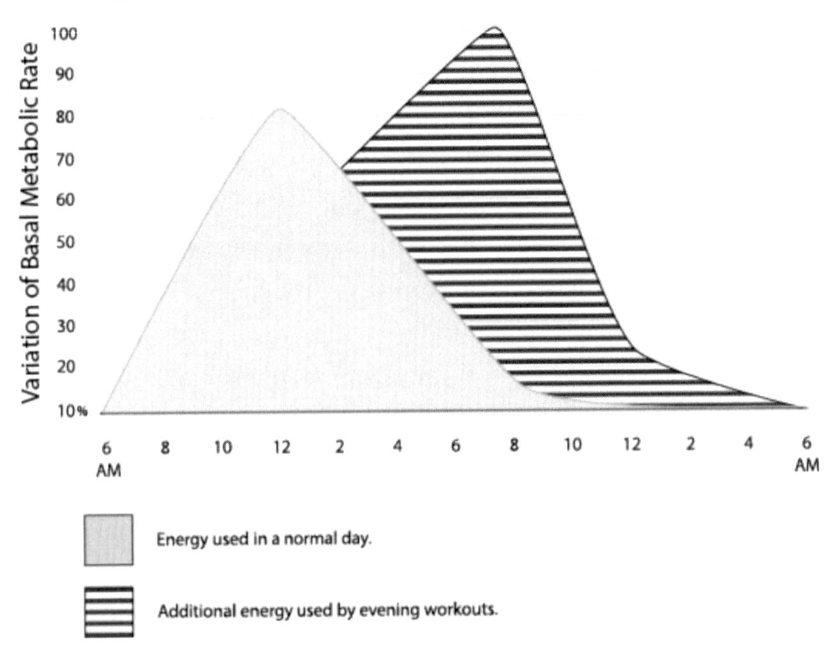

CHAPTER SEVEN

Tendonosis

The Most Misdiagnosed Musculoskeletal Condition

A musculoskeletal condition is any condition that relates to the frame of the body and its moving parts; for example, bone, cartilage, ligaments, muscles, and tendons. Before we discuss injuries and treatment in the next chapter, I think it's time to give you the goods on this common problem. You might wonder why I dedicated an entire chapter to a condition you may never have heard of. Tendonosis is often referred to as "tendinopathy" and mistakenly called "tendinitis." Most doctors misdiagnose tendonosis as tendinitis. In this chapter, I'm going to explain how to tell one from the other. Understanding the difference will save you months of pain and a lot of cash at your doctor or physical therapist's office. After reading this short chapter, you will be able to recognize and treat this condition without the help of any doctors. For the purposes of explanation, we will use elbow tendonosis in this chapter. Chapter 9 will deal with several injuries, including tendonosis problems at other parts of the body.

Tendinitis

When young people hurt a tendon, either through trauma or repetitive use, the tendon suffers small tears and gets inflamed. Plain and simple, tendinitis is an inflammation of the tendon. Inflammation is the number one way our bodies send pain messages to our brain. Treating elbow tendinitis with ice, anti-inflammatory medication, and counter bracing (**wolfelbowbrace.com**) should manage this condition quite nicely. The time that it takes to recover from tendinitis differentiates it from tendonosis. If a person is over 35 and the elbow is not better in 6 weeks, they probably don't have tendinitis – they have tendonosis.

Tendonosis

As discussed in Chapters 4 and 5, the connective tissue in the body loses water content as it ages. This phenomenon accounts for microscopic tears in the matrix of the tendon fibers. As tissue ages, it also loses blood flow. This decreased vascularity, coupled with dehydration, accounts for the slow death of the tissue. This starts to happen in our mid-30s. Basically, aging tendons are degenerating and dying. When operating on a healthy tendon, the surgeon will note a nice white matrix of the tendon body. However, tendinopathy (a degenerated tendon) will look gray. Having lost water and vascularity, this tissue is now more brittle than it was originally. This fragility results in cracks that lead to inflammation – and inflammation means pain.

The elbow is one of the most common places to experience this injury. If affected on the outside of the elbow, it's called "tennis elbow." If occurring on the inside of the elbow, it's called "bowler's elbow." If you're over 35 and have been diagnosed with tennis elbow or some other tendon injury that won't heal, you probably have tendonosis.

Differences Between Tendinits And Tendonosis

Compared to tendonosis, tendinitis responds well to rest and bracing. Unfortunately, tendonosis gets worse with rest and needs to be treated. The good news here is that I am going to tell you how to get rid of tendinitis and tendonosis for good.

Not long ago, you would go to the doctor and get diagnosed with tennis elbow tendinitis and would be told to rest it. If you didn't do anything for a month or two, the elbow might start to feel better, but as soon as you pick up a heavy object or shake someone's hand, the pain would shoot back. The tennis elbow brace, also known as a counter brace (**wolfelbowbrace.com**), helps tremendously to reduce the pressure on the elbow and thereby the pain. A brace like this and/or a support that provides compression, coupled with The Big Five (which I will discuss in Chapter 8), are generally all that is needed for treating tendinitis. When suffering tendonosis, however, the pain comes back as soon as the counter brace is removed. Frustrated, you returned to your doctor, who would send you to an orthopedist that then diagnosed you with a stubborn case. The orthopedist would give you a cortisone shot that might have helped with the pain but in fact could have worsened the tendinopathy. A few shots later, the doctors would decide to operate, cutting the tendon away from the bone and reattaching it, with a couple of months of physical therapy to follow. Basically, the surgery performed forced the body to rebuild the decaying tissue. The next section will show you how to avoid surgery.

How To Fix Tendonosis Without Surgery

Here's how to get rid of tendonosis in a few weeks. The key thought here is we want to stimulate the body to rebuild itself without chopping you up with a surgical procedure. To do this, we need to put a tension load into the tendon. In essence, this will force the body to rebuild.

There are two types of tension forces we can put into the tendon. A concentric force is a positive force or a force that shortens the tendon and muscle. Concentric forces are lifting forces. This force is what happens during the act of curling a weight. Concentric exercise is good for building muscle, but not rebuilding tendons.

Eccentric force is the exact opposite of concentric force. Eccentric force is a negative force. They lengthen the tendon and muscle. These forces are lowering forces.

This eccentric stress causes disruption of the tendon matrix. Basically, we are making a small injury to the tissue. We want to stimulate activity in the tendon in an effort to force the body to completely rebuild the structure. I suggest using this negative force in 2-second increments. I have videos at my website **DrDeanWolf.com**, that show how to do this. But for now, let's stick with good old tennis elbow. Here's how to treat it. For example's sake, let's say we are suffering from lateral epicondylitis (tennis elbow) of the right elbow. You could take a light dumbbell – anywhere from 5-15 lbs – and hold it up with your right hand as the following picture shows.

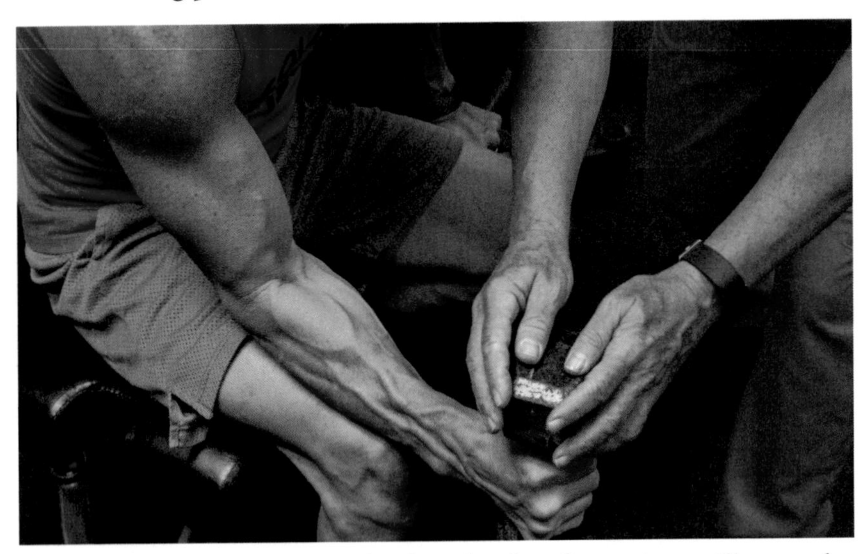

Then your left hand, or the hand of a therapist, will cup the top of the dumbbell, and pull the dumbbell inward. (A counterclockwise movement when looking at the dumbbell.) This movement should take 2 full seconds to achieve 90° of motion. Simultaneously, while doing this inward pull, your right hand is resisting the motion. You will feel pain over the outside of your right elbow. I'm not going to lie to you, this freakin' hurts!

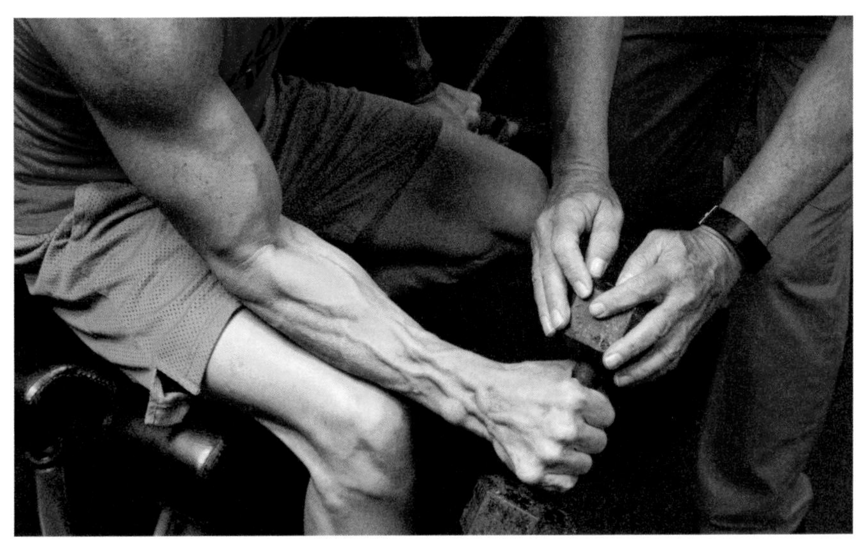

We should do 4 sets of 15 repetitions with these 2-second periods of resistance. Some experts say do them every day. I found doing them every other day is torture enough. Almost every case I've treated is cured in 4-6 weeks. If you are unsure of this procedure, go to **DrDeanWolf.com** to watch videos demonstrating how simple this is to do.

I remember getting tennis elbow in my mid-40s and performing this routine. The first 2-3 times I absolutely dreaded the thought of it – but here's the cool part. I saw immediate changes for the better. The very first time doing the routine, I noticed that I had serious pain during every repetition on all 4 sets. However, I did notice during the last couple reps of the final set that the pain wasn't as severe. The next time, I felt just mild discomfort on the last few reps of the final set. After about 10 days, I barely had any discomfort on the last set. Then, after another week, I had even less pain in the third set. And so on and so forth. The tendonosis-affected area gets better quickly and it helps keep a person motivated when they see progress. The challenge is just to grin and bear it for the first couple of times.

In the last 10 years, I've personally experienced tendonosis in five different body parts. I had it in the inner and outer part of my right elbow. I've also had it in the bicep of my right arm. I've had it in front of my knee over the patellar tendon. Lastly, it occurred in my right biceps femoris (hamstring). With each of these injuries, I performed 4 sets of 15 repetitions with negative force for 2-second holds every other day for about 4-6 weeks. I had complete resolution. The point being, as we get older, we can rebuild these used parts with a little know-how. Getting old ain't for the faint of heart.

CHAPTER EIGHT

Spinal Injury, Prevention and Treatment

Beds

I decided to discuss beds in the beginning of this chapter because it's so important for spine health to sleep on the right type of surface. One of the most commonly asked questions in my clinical setting is, "What kind of bed should I have?" Fundamentally, you need to make sure you don't sleep in a position that makes your spine bow in any direction. Selecting the type of mattress that achieves this is not so simple and here's why. Three factors determine what type of bed you should have. First, all of us are shaped differently. Second, we have different body mass or weight. Third, sleep position can play a role in mattress choice. Let's take these one at a time.

1) Body Shape

The key to ensuring that you don't wake up with back pain is to sleep in a way that does not compromise the spine. You have to make sure that there is balance regarding your body position.

For example, if you lay on your side, you want your spine to be straight.

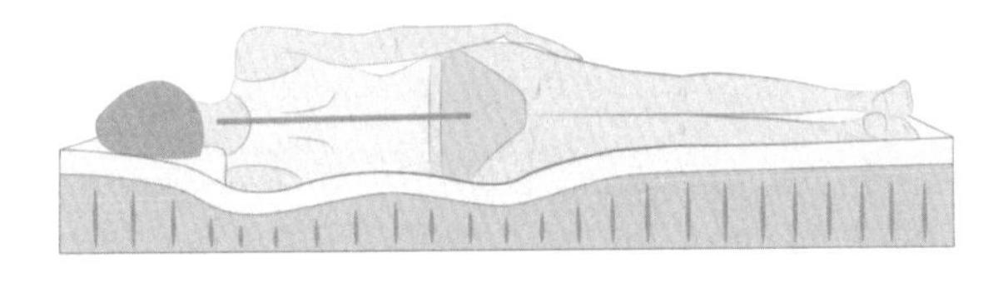

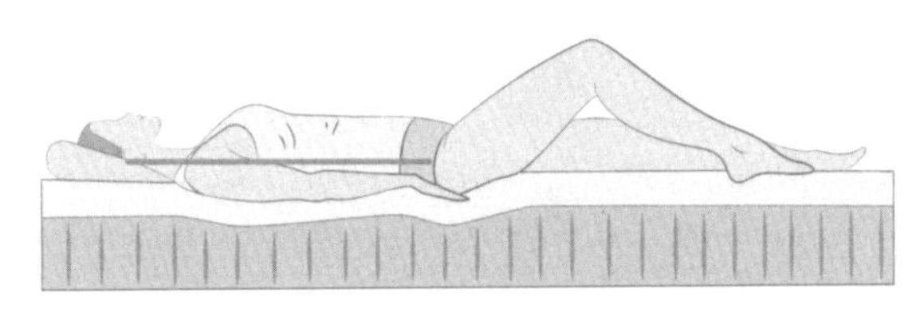

Your body shape can dictate what type of mattress will be most able to support you in this position. If you have large hips, similar to typical female anatomy, you might need a softer mattress to absorb your body contours. If you are a man with very wide shoulders, the same could be true.The same holds true if you are a back sleeper and have a curvy body shape. You would want a mattress on the softer side to absorb your body's natural curves. Conversely, if you have a flatter body shape and you sleep on your back or side on a soft mattress, you will "sink" into the mattress, creating a bowing effect and thus increasing the chance of waking up with back pain. As seen on the following three diagrams.

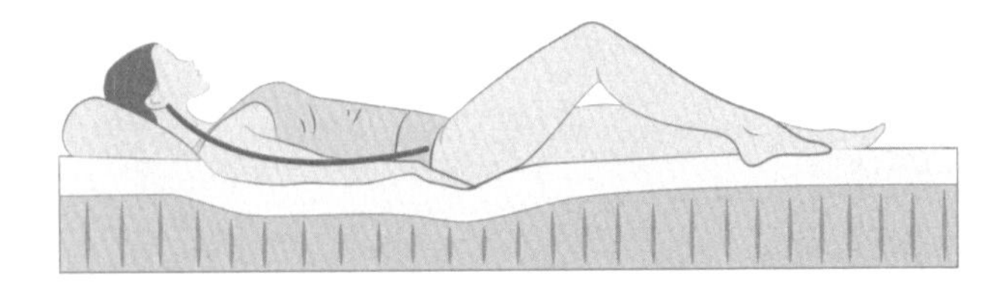

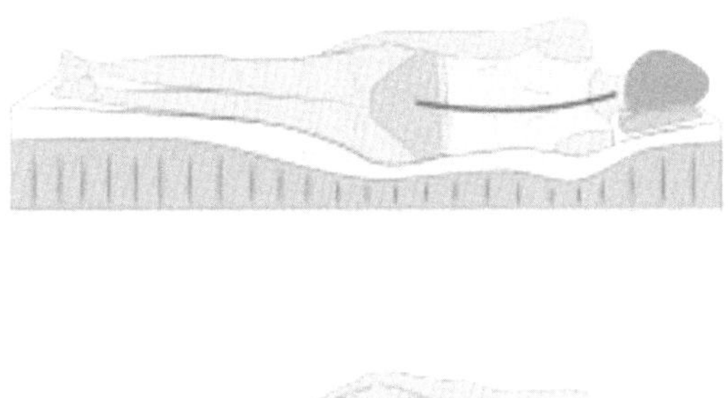

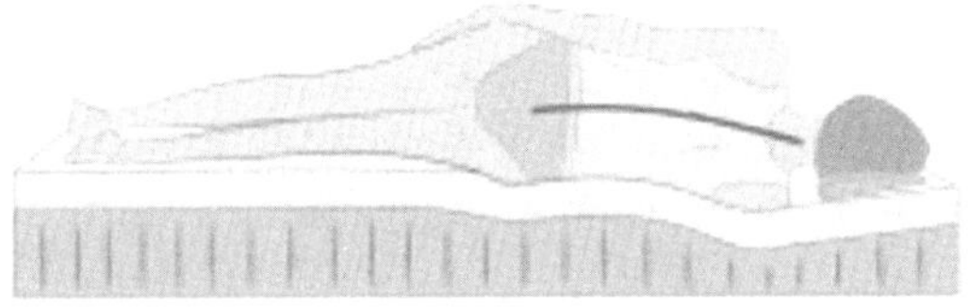

Body Mass

A heavy person will "sink" into a mattress more than a lighter person. It's pure physics. In general, a heavier person should have a firmer mattress and a lighter person should have a softer mattress. Back problems arise when there is a couple sleeping on the same "surface," with one person being much heavier than the other. This is clearly an instance when each person needs to be on a different mattress with appropriate firmness. In these cases, the couple should select a bed that has firmness settings that can be adjusted from one side to the other to compensate for the different body masses. A nice trick to making one side of your bed firmer is to cut a piece of plywood and place it between the mattress and box spring.

Body Position

Sleep position adds an entirely different dynamic to determining the type of mattress you should have. We just discussed body shape and mass and their role in selecting the right mattress. If you have very wide hips and you are a "side sleeper," you will want to sleep on a softer mattress. But if you have wide hips, are a "back sleeper," don't have a curvy rear end, and aren't heavy, you will want to sleep on a firmer mattress. Once again, the key is to avoid bowing of your spine as you sleep.

Lastly, never sleep on your stomach. If you sleep on your side, avoid any twisted positions. When sleeping on your side, you will find putting a pillow between your legs can help stabilize you from rolling or twisting your lower back while sleeping.

The Big Five

This chapter is going to deal with common spinal problems that people age 40-plus typically encounter. We will discuss the most common disorders and injuries, how to prevent them, and how to treat them. This chapter can be considered a reference guide. You can skip to the conditions that interest you and bypass the others. If you don't have one of the conditions mentioned herein, you might later and you can reference this text as needed. If you suffer from one of these afflictions, reading over the particulars will be of more interest to you. There will be no Nuts and Bolts section in this chapter. If the spinal problem does not pertain to you, just skip to the next subject. In effect, the entire chapter is a Nuts and Bolts read.

I have found success treating spinal injuries using a combination of five different procedures. Let's call this the "Big Five." This multi-tier approach consists of: 1) icing; 2) anti-inflammatory medications; 3) physical forms of medicine, like EMS (Electric Muscle Stimulation), ultrasound, and mechanical traction; 4) chiropractic care; and 5) nutritional support. Almost all the conditions and injuries in this chapter respond well to the Big Five. So, let's identify them one by one.

1) Ice

Icing is extremely effective in the treatment of all orthopedic injuries. It still amazes me how many doctors will put heat on a joint. I am convinced that the only reason heat modalities are used in formal therapy settings is because the insurance company reimbursements are higher for heat than cold. I could do an entire chapter on ICE VS. HEAT. Simply put, all the things that heat brings to the table, ice does better. Heat expands tissue and should not be put over joints. The only use for heat I can see is in a controlled therapy setting, in order to expand injured muscle tissue before performing stretching routines. On the other hand, ice constricts the tissue, which can disperse the edema (swelling) out of the injured site. Swelling takes up space, which creates pressure. This consequential pressure is what pain is all about. Reduce pressure and you will reduce pain. I have been practicing chiropractic for over 30 years. On average, I have seen forty to fifty patients a day. A day never goes by that I don't hear a patient tell me, "My back hurt a little last night and I put a heating pad on it and it felt better, then this morning I woke up and couldn't move. I don't know if I slept funny or what." If you take an inflamed area and put heat on it, the condition will worsen.

Another benefit of ice is that when the human body senses the cold, its innate thermostatic intelligence kicks in. You see, one of the reasons our body regulates temperature is so chemical reactions occur at certain rates of speed. The higher the temperature, the faster the process proceeds. That's why fever occurs when we are sick. The higher the temperature, the faster the body works to get rid of the bug. With the exception of any fever over 104°F, fever is good. Since every tissue heals proportionally to its blood supply, anything we can do to get more blood flowing to bring nutrients to the tissue will help it heal faster. Ever notice the big red mark on your skin after you remove ice? This big red mark is a function of the vasoconstriction vasodilation reflex. Ice reduces swelling and, at the same time, tricks the body into sending more blood to warm the tissue to avoid damage. We can use this phenomenon to help injuries heal quicker. More blood equals shorter recovery times. Ligaments have small amounts of blood flow, resulting in longer recovery periods. Tendons have more vascularity than ligaments but not as much as muscles. Muscles have large amounts of blood flow and therefore shorter recovery times. Ice also has a numbing effect. Ice will decrease pain, and as far as I'm concerned, there is no valor in suffering.

Here's the only caveat with ice. Never leave the ice on longer than 20 minutes. The first 20 minutes achieve a push of water out of the tissue, reducing swelling and pain. If ice is left on the skin longer than 20 minutes, you could get some skin damage. Also after 20 minutes, the body's thermal protection instinct kicks in and it will do anything to warm up the area, including sending water. Lymphatic constriction occurs after 20 minutes of ice. This is trouble, because your lymph system is what carries the swelling or edema away from the injured site. Lymphatic constriction decreases this drainage, which is not good – we don't want any further swelling. The goal here is to achieve the vasoconstriction vasodilation reflex. With ice, you want to get in and get out, get in and get out. We want to make the body bring more blood in and carry swelling out. A good treatment regimen would be to ice 20 minutes every hour on the hour. I like this best because two things get accomplished. I can keep track of when I put the ice on, and the 40 minutes off gives my ice pack time to recharge in the freezer. If you want to be aggressive with your ice treatment, you can ice 20 minutes on and 20 minutes off. You will need more than one ice pack for this. The ice packs I use are the ones that have a soft cloth outside covering which prevents ice burn on the skin.

2) Anti-Inflammatory Medication

Prostaglandins are the chemicals our bodies produce to bring about inflammation and pain. This is a natural defense mechanism created in an effort to make you guard or protect an injured area. The problem with this process, in addition to said pain and inflammation, is that it ultimately slows down your recovery time. Nonsteroidal anti-inflammatory drugs (NSAIDs) are useful in blocking prostaglandin production. These products can be purchased over the counter. This includes aspirin, ibuprofen, and naproxen. The differences are based on the time of action. Aspirin works effectively for 4 hours, ibuprofen for 8 hours, and naproxen for 12 hours. Using these weapons helps attack pain and decreases recovery time by lowering the swelling. There are prescription NSAIDs that have 24 hours of action. Common ones include Celebrex, Mobic, and Vioxx. The biggest problem with NSAIDs is that they can irritate the lining of the stomach. No matter how good your stomach is, I recommend buffering the NSAID with some food. Of the over-the-counter NSAIDs, I prefer naproxen because of its longer acting capability. When you're going through the acute phase of injury, it's best to take NSAIDs systematically every day. I recommend taking them for up to 2-4 weeks to reduce swelling and to allow the body to heal.

3) Physical Medicine

EMS, ultrasound, mechanical traction, and massage are great forms of physical medicine. These modalities are ways of creating metabolic activity or physiology. You basically speed up the body's chemistry through disruption. The art of physical medicine is to irritate the body enough to stimulate an increase in vascular response without causing physical damage, effectively forcing the body to heal quicker than it would on its own. There's a reason physical therapists and chiropractors alike have been using them for years. They work!

EMS is "electric muscle stimulation" and is great for relaxing the muscle tissue and increasing blood flow to it. EMS can be used over ligaments and tendons, too. The mechanical disruption via electric signals promotes dispersal of swelling in injured tissue. This modality also has a short-term numbing effect that can help manage pain. There are several types of EMS that include High Voltage Stimulation, Interferential Current, Iontophoresis, Neuromuscular Electrical Stimulation, and Russian Stimulation. These forms of electric muscle stimulation are performed in supervised clinical settings. TENS is "transcutaneous electrical nerve stimulation." This form of EMS is used to help manage pain. The way this works is through the principle of synaptic fatigue. Synaptic fatigue might be best explained metaphorically. Consider a visit to a dairy farm. At first, you smell the unpleasant odor of cow manure. After a short period of time, you become desensitized and don't notice the smell. Through the use of a TENS unit, we are able to help reduce pain by using the same physiologic principles. When applying continuous, low-voltage stimulation to an area of injury, your brain stops noticing the electrical sensation after a few minutes; along with that, your body stops noticing the pain, too. I have found these units to be very helpful in managing pain. Drawing from 30 years of clinical experience, I specifically designed a TENS unit that has a convenient touch screen with settings to manage both acute and chronic pain. The unit is rechargeable so you won't have to keep buying 9-volt batteries (**wolftensunit.com**).

Ultrasound therapy uses high frequency sound waves to promote blood flow and help break up adhesions on a microscopic level. Ultrasound increases membrane permeability, allowing for more cellular transport. This helps the injured site heal quicker. Additionally, ultrasound is the deepest penetrating modality. The sound waves can penetrate 4-8 centimeters, making this form of therapy helpful in treating deep tissue injury. Since ultrasound stimulates the release of endorphins, it is helpful with pain control. This modality has been around since 1940, the reason being that it really works.

When it comes to disc protrusions in the neck or low back, mechanical traction or flexion distraction are effective in creating a nuclear migration of the disc. By physically distracting the protrusion, it helps the disc to regain its normal position. The movement of the bulge back to the center of the disc is called nuclear migration. This movement is another way we can "disrupt" the body to help stimulate activity, resulting in shorter recovery times. Think of nuclear migration like this: if you take a piece of paper that is bulging and pull it apart, or "distract it," the protrusion is removed.

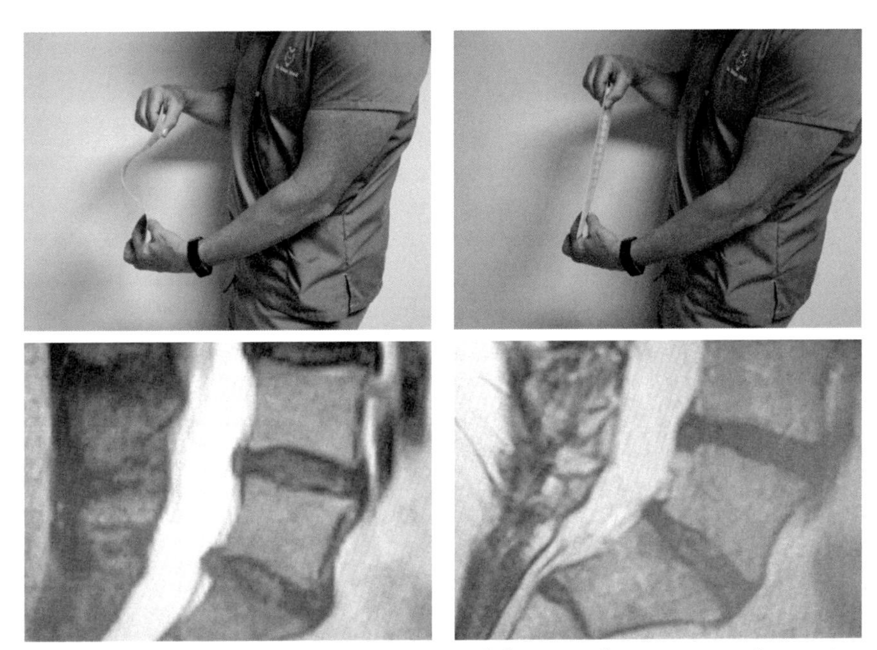

And that is exactly how traction and flexion distraction therapies work.

4) Chiropractic Care

One of the most useful things chiropractors do, wittingly or not, is restore motion. One of the problems with injuries that include disc herniations and protrusions, fixed joints and subluxations, as well as strains and sprains alike, is that the surrounding tissue becomes fibrotic and locks up in an effort to "cast" the injured area. The problem with this response is that it takes up space, vis-a-vis swelling. Also, scar tissue forms from lack of movement. By inducing motion into the corresponding joints, movement is restored, scar tissue is broken up, and vascularity is stimulated. When the bones are in their proper juxtaposition, normal mechanics can take place with ease. Manual adjustments into areas with disc herniations are potentially harmful, so you want a chiropractor to perform any manipulative therapy – they are highly trained in this art. Specific manipulation is key. Short-lever induced motion will be less likely to produce further injury or pain than long-lever gross manipulation. Short-lever adjusting techniques are taught at chiropractic universities. Long-lever techniques are antiquated and potentially harmful but are still performed by untrained therapists. Long-lever techniques can cause shear into the soft tissue component of the injured area, especially discs. These are the manipulative techniques that you see on those YouTube videos where a person is cracking every bone in someone's body. Here is an example of a long-lever technique.

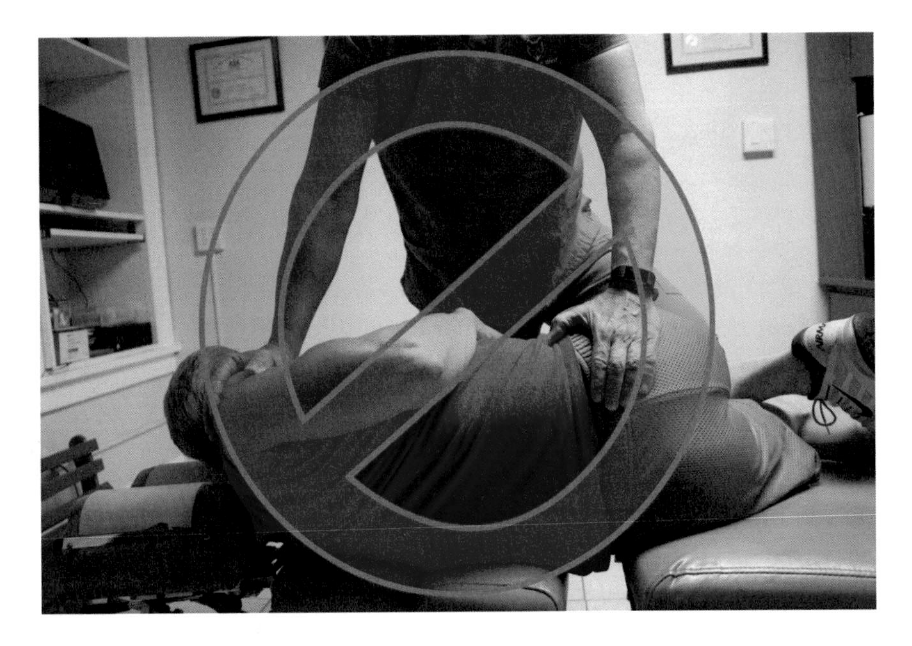

Notice the chiropractor's right hand is on the patient's shoulder and the left hand is on the patient's hip. This technique is "old school" and predisposes the patient to injury from the excess twisting motion. The following picture shows a "short-lever" technique that differentiates chiropractors from other health care doctors that perform manipulative medicine.

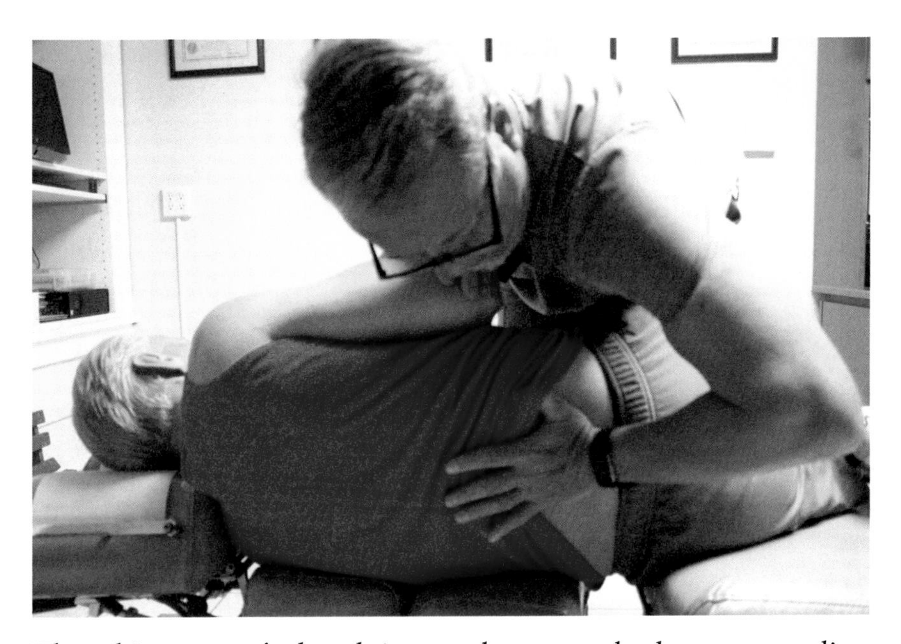

The chiropractor's hand is on the exact body part needing adjusting, pushing in a specific line of correction. Short-lever techniques are targeted methods that decrease chance of patient injury. There's a reason you see a chiropractor on every block. They know what they are doing. When done correctly, chiropractic procedures are extremely therapeutic for all injuries, including disc injuries.

5) Nutritional Support

Supporting injured structures with certain supplements can be helpful. I'm a big believer in glucosamine sulfate in combination with chondroitin and MSM for joint nutritional support (**wolfjointrebuild.com**). Type II collagen helps provide the proteins the body uses to help rebuild connective tissue. Turmeric and ginger have been clearly found to have anti-inflammatory capabilities. If you're looking to try this supplement, we have a good one on my website (**wolftumeric.com**). Blueberries and other natural berries have phytonutrients that can help reduce inflammation and pain. Even avocados have been found to have anti-inflammatory nutrients. Resveratrol, which is found in red wine, can quiet down inflammation. Omega-3 fatty acids (wolfomega3.com) have been shown to have similar effects to that of Celebrex, the COX 2 inhibitor, that is prescribed for inflammation.

Regarding the Big Five treatment, I think it's reasonable to try all of these in a shotgun approach. Sometimes any one treatment on its own will not be the proverbial silver bullet. The patient that uses more of these weapons will heal faster than the patient that uses only one or two. Now let's discuss specific spinal problems.

Cervical Spine Problems

Injury to the cervical spine is commonplace in the gym. Once again, as we age the connective tissue loses water and this dehydration process makes the tissue susceptible to cracks and fissures. A healthy cervical spine has a lordotic curve. This curve increases the mechanical strength of the structures of the neck. Loss of this curve, or even worse, reversal of this curve geometrically increases your chance of injury. The basic premise of maintaining this cervical curve, like wearing an orthotic for the foot, is the backdrop of preventing a multitude of neck injuries, especially while we are exercising.

Basically, there are three main cervical components that will get compromised in a gym environment: the disc, the facet joint, and the small muscles of the neck. Tendon and ligament injuries can occur, too, but they aren't as common and are usually the result of some sort of trauma, like a car accident. Let's take each of these components one at a time.

A) Discs

Discs are the connective tissue that sit in between the vertebral bones in the neck. Discs are often referred to as "spacers" or "cushions between the bones." There's a perception with this terminology that they are soft or maybe weak. This couldn't be farther from the truth. The discs are extremely strong fibrocartilage. In fact, the disc is stronger than the bone. The reason being, the disc is mostly water. Water is more dense than bone. Because discs have such a high water content, the discs are tough mothers. The disc has two basic components to it: an outside covering called the annulus fibrosus and inside component called the nucleus pulposus.

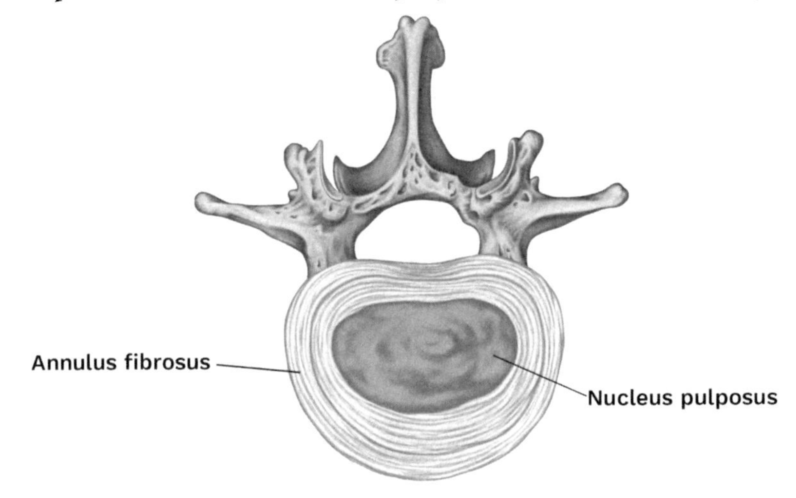

NORMAL DISC

The annulus of the disc reminds me of a steel-belted radial tire. In fact, I think the inventors of that tire stole its design from Mother Nature. The fibers are oblique in nature and traverse each other. This makes for an incredibly strong matrix.

The nucleus pulposus of the disc is like the inner tube of a tire. It's mostly made of water, acts as a shock absorber for the spine, and maintains space between the vertebrae.

The disc is extremely strong against compressive forces. In fact, the bone will break before the disc does. However, the disc is vulnerable to oblique, shear-type forces. So, a twisting-while-lifting motion is a prescription for blowing out a disc. Snow shoveling, lifting heavy things out of a trunk of a car, and even a golf swing, to some degree, can create this type of shear. When the outside of the disc gets a tear, the outward nuclear pressure from the center of the disc creates a bulge in the disc.

Because of the proximity of the spinal cord and nerve structures, the body has a particularly vicious inflammatory response to this injury site. Space is of the essence in the body and especially around the spinal cord. So any "space-occupying" lesion, whether it be the bulge of the disc itself or the swelling, creates pressure. Pressure receptors (baroreceptors) report to your brain that you have pain. The only good thing about getting old is the fact that as we age the disc starts to lose its size. As it shrinks, it's less likely to create a space occupying lesion. Because of this, disc issues will be more problematic in your 30s and 40s than your 50s and 60s.

My favorite clinical analogy regarding the mechanism of disc protrusions is as follows. When I was a child, I had this bike that had an old tire. The tire was dry rotted, which isn't too far from what happens to our tissues as we age. The sidewalls of the tire had big, gaping cracks, and I could see its inner tube. I'd take my air pump and inflate the tire so much that the inner tube would bulge out of the sidewall. This is exactly what happens with a herniated disc. The nucleus pulposus will protrude outside of the containment of the annulus. This is a true herniation.

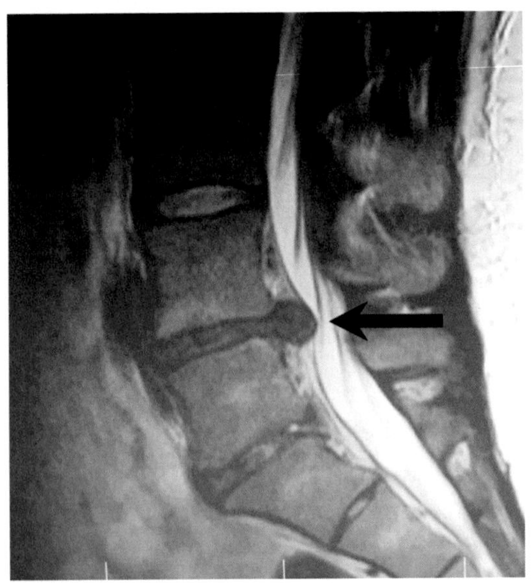

Once this injury rears its ugly head, it's a continual problem for us geriatric athletes. When the normal cervical curve is maintained, the anatomy is designed to have a natural, mechanical form of protection. The natural, mechanical force pushes the disc to the anterior, or front of the spine. This is good because the ligament that runs down the front of the spine is thick and super strong, like steel. Absent severe trauma, the disc usually won't herniate out the front of the neck. Not to mention, there are no nerve structures directly in front of the neck. Conversely, you can see by the following X-rays that a reverse curve predisposes protrusion forces to the posterior, or back of the spine. Just as if you were to press on the front of a peanut butter and jelly sandwich the jelly would be pushed out the back. The same principle holds true when your neck is in mechanical compromise with a reversed curve.

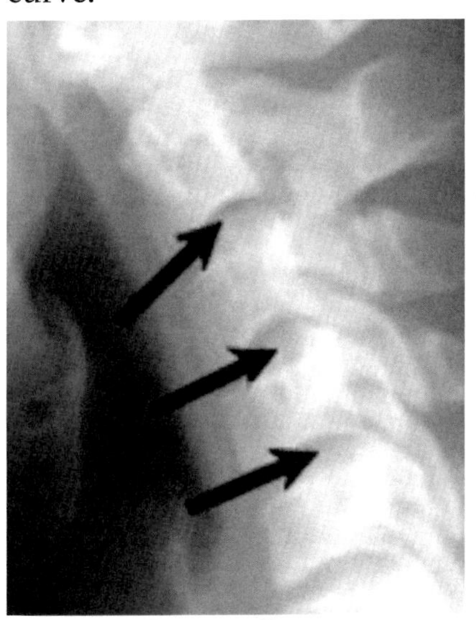

Reverse Curve

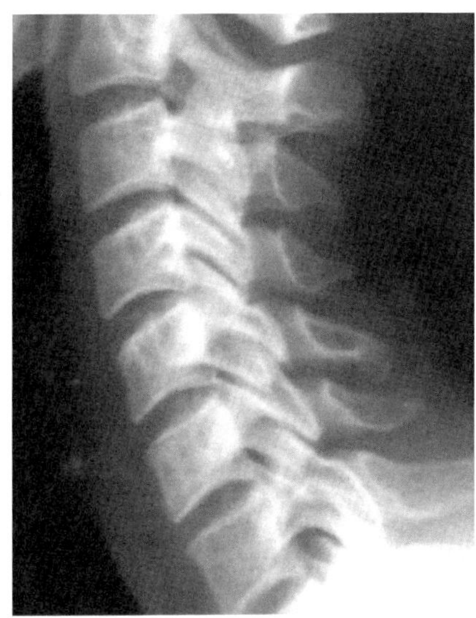

Normal Curve

The ligament in the back of the spinal column is called the posterior longitudinal ligament. This ligament is smaller and isn't completely able to contain disc protrusion forces. Worst of all, this is where all the neural structures are. Maintaining the cervical curve during exercise is paramount in reducing the likelihood of neck injury. The picture on the following page shows how any exercise on a bench puts one in a position where the cervical curve is reduced.

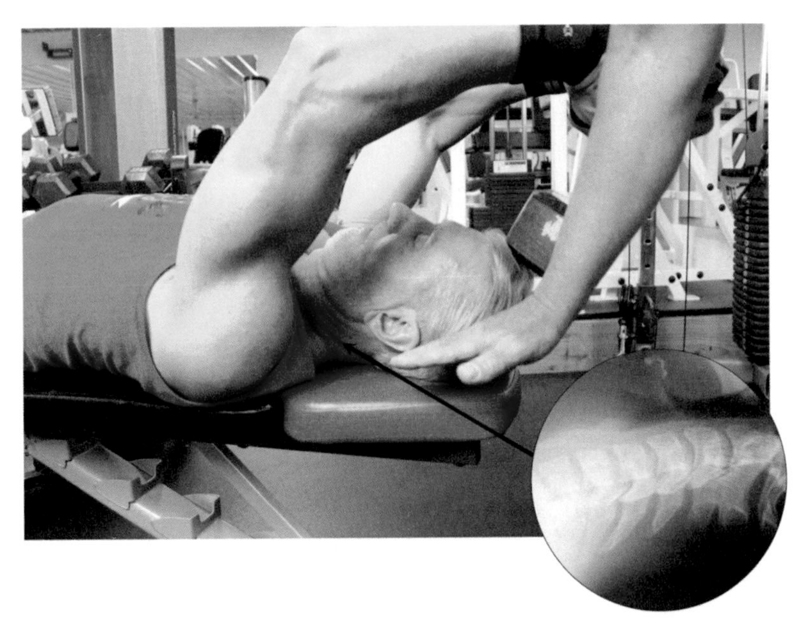

The next picture shows how simply putting a pillow or rolled up towel under your neck can protect its natural curve during exercises that involve lying on your back.

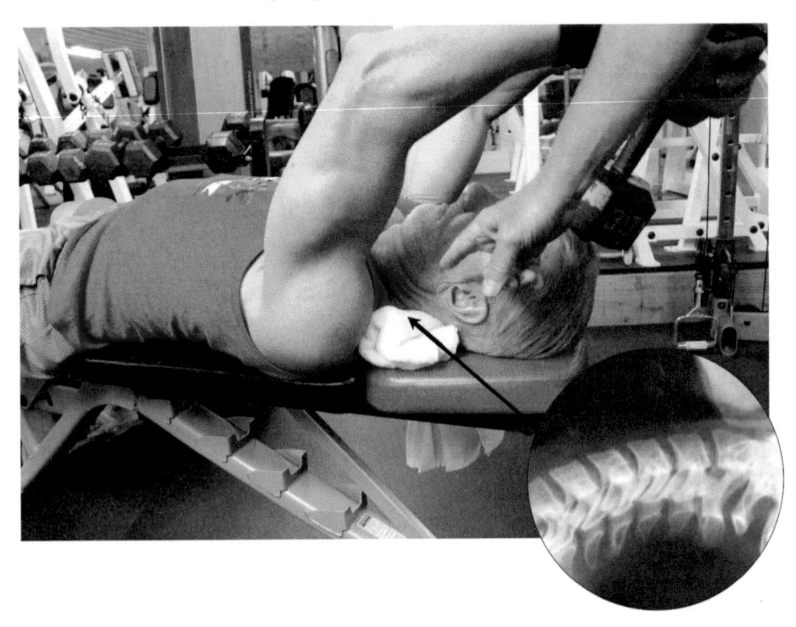

Another way of protecting your neck from injury is to maintain a solid posture when doing pulling exercises. Just simple movement of the shoulders to the front creates a slight loss of neck curve. So, if you have the dreaded "bad posture" or posterior shoulder instability problems, you should make sure your shoulders are back while exercising. Consciously holding your shoulders back during lat pulls, for example, protects your neck quite nicely. The following picture on the left shows a forward position of the shoulders and therefore a bad technique. On the right is a better technique with the shoulders slightly back, helping to maintain the natural cervical curve.

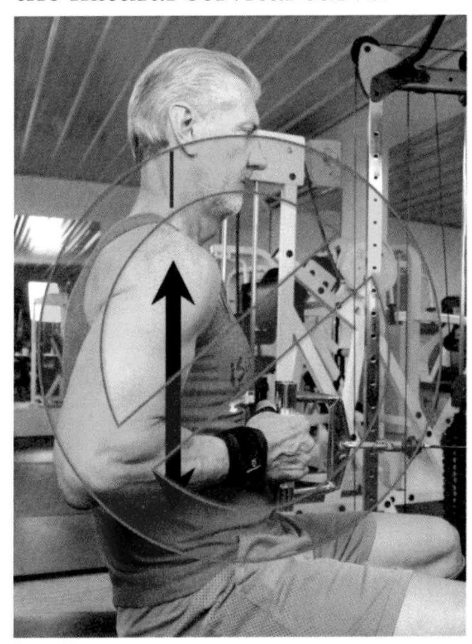

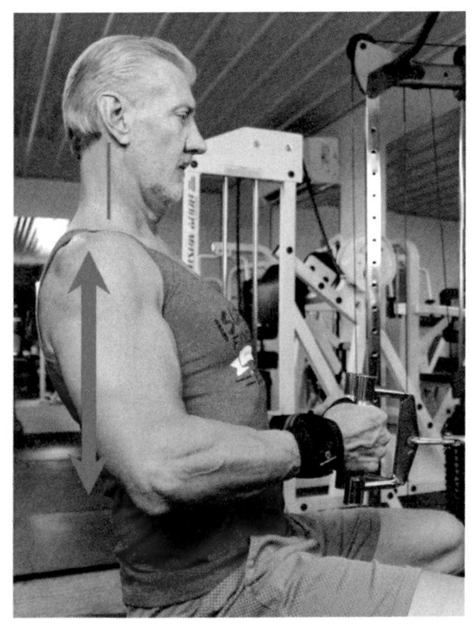

Treating neck disc injuries with the Big Five is quite effective, particularly with mechanical traction. If you have a chronic neck disc issue, you should buy yourself a home traction unit and use it several times a week. Mechanical distraction helps facilitate nuclear migration of the disc protrusion. A TENS unit can help with chronic pain, especially pain at night (**wolftensunit.com**).

If there is pain down the arm (radicular pain), it could be due to massive swelling, for which a prescribed corticosteroid pack might help. Epidural steroid injections from a pain management specialist can help with the most difficult cases. If you have pain that radiates down the arm, you must be evaluated by a chiropractor, neurosurgeon or orthopedic surgeon right away.

Surgical intervention might be required if there is a severe herniation.

B) Cervical Strains and Sprains of the Facet Joint

Facets are joints that connect one bone to another in the neck. These joints sit like shingles on a roof. Once again, maintaining the normal cervical curve protects these facets from strain. When the neck loses its lordotic curve or when your head is put in flexion, the facet joint is vulnerable to strain.

The same principles for protecting facets from injury hold true for protecting discs from injury. Maintaining a normal lordosis while exercising will prevent strains from occurring.

Treatments for facet injuries are almost identical to those of disc injuries. Ice is probably the most important because reducing swelling in a joint is priority number one when it comes to recovery. NSAIDs are helpful too. Treatment for a facet injury is where chiropractic care stands out. Maintaining vertebral alignment and keeping normal joint motion is so important during recovery. Nutritional support is also useful, just as with disc injuries.

C) Muscles

Muscle injury in the neck most commonly occurs with the small muscles. The large muscles of the neck are usually injured by trauma. When injuring a small muscle in the neck, rest is probably the most underrated treatment approach. These small muscles have lots of blood flow and heal quickly when not continually reinjured. I've found that many patients have difficulty recovering from neck muscle injuries because they've induced trauma into the area before it's completely recovered. Ice and NSAIDs help tremendously.

Thoracic Spine Problems

Because the anatomy of the middle back (thoracic spine) is different from the cervical area, there is a variety of injuries that can take place. The thoracic spine has a kyphotic curve. This curve is the exact opposite of the cervical and lumbar spine.

Thoracic strains and subluxations are common. Compression fractures occur more in this part of the back than in other areas of the spine. Intercostal strains, costochondritis, and rib subluxations can be seen, too. Disc injuries in the thoracic spine are unusual. The structure of the thoracic spine is more stable than the cervical and lumbar spine. The ribs and extensive back muscles make the thoracic spine's range of motion limited in comparison to the neck and lower back. This decreased range of motion reduces the likelihood of injuries.

A) Thoracic Strains and Subluxations

Thoracic strains are a result of excess stress placed on the soft tissue connections to the thoracic spine. These strains can be to the capsule of the joint or the muscle or tendon connecting the joint. Typically, we don't see as many strains in the middle back as we do in the neck and lower back. This is primarily due to less range of motion. When doing weight training, it's important to maintain stable body mechanics.

Additionally, the more rest someone gets, the more likely soft tissues can recover. Sleeping on your back or side is helpful in preventing back strains; however, sleeping on your stomach puts a mechanical load of stress on the facet joints. This extra stress results in less rest and recovery for the joint, thereby predisposing you to injury.

Treatment for thoracic strains is primarily rest. These tissues recover fast because of their vascularity and their proximity to the heart. EMS and ultrasound work great for helping to promote increased blood flow. As you know, you can't go wrong with ice. Subluxation or fixation of the joint responds well to chiropractic care.

B) Thoracic Compression Fractures

Compression fractures are most common in the thoracic spine and occur in women more than men. The primary cause of these fractures is osteoporosis. These fractures are seen mostly in the lower thoracic spine but can occur anywhere. If you have ever seen a very old person that was bent forward with a large humpback, chances are you are looking at someone that has had one or more compression fractures. When the vertebrae collapses, it usually occurs in the front of the vertebrae. This creates a wedge effect and is responsible for the humpback appearance.

Other causes of compression fractures are the demineralization of bone from certain medications like long-term prednisone use. Another cause is pathology. Cancers spread to the bone, causing erosion to the point where it collapses. Lastly, trauma can play a causal role in suffering a compression fracture.

Treatment typically includes rest and back bracing to limit movement and reduce pain. NSAIDs can help as well as ice. Surgical treatment via kyphoplasty and vertebroplasty have come a long way. Kyphoplasty uses balloons to inflate the vertebrae to its normal height, then vertebroplasty is performed to keep the bone there. With vertebroplasty, a specially formulated acrylic cement is injected into the collapsed vertebrae in an effort to stabilize the bone from further collapse. This reduces pain and also provides a cosmetic improvement in the patient's posture. It can tremendously improve the patient's ability to stand erect.

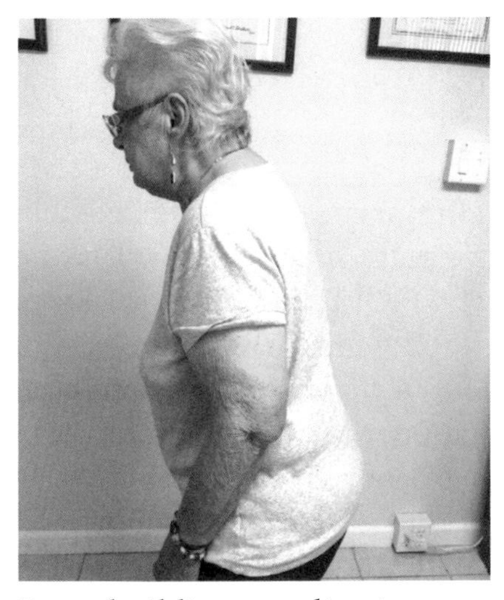
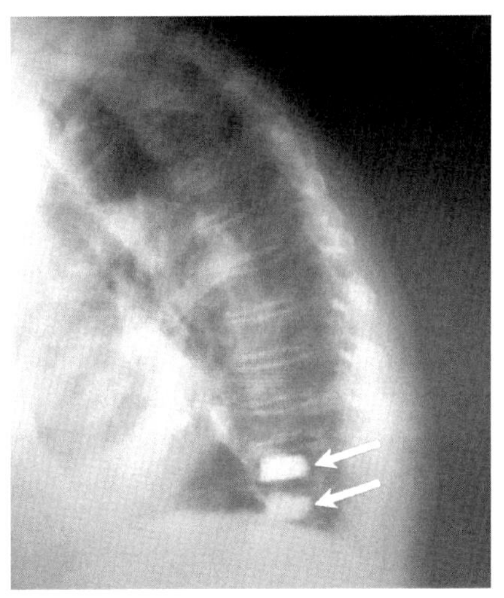

Bone-building medications and hormone therapy can help prevent osteoporosis. If you're osteoporotic, you need to have a bone density test and complete hormone work-up to see if there's a primary, treatable reason for the loss of bone. Everyone over age 50 should take a calcium supplement with vitamin D to support bone health (**wolfbonebuild.com**).

C) Costochondritis, Intercostal Strains, and Rib Subluxations

Costochondritis or chest wall pain might not necessarily have a known cause. This occurs when inflammation strikes the cartilage that connects the ribs to the sternum. This condition is painful and quite disconcerting because of the chest pain associated with it. This injury makes it difficult to work out. However, you could probably do cardio training with this injury without too much difficulty.

Intercostal strains can occur more frequently as we age. The tissue between the ribs can lose water like all the other structures in our body. As a result, there's less elasticity when bending and twisting.

Rib dislocations (subluxations) can occur with any activity, even something as benign as a cough or sneeze. This condition is extremely painful. Anyone that's had this one really appreciates a good chiropractor. Usually, the reduction of the rib subluxation gives instant relief.

Treatment of all three of these conditions consists of management of symptoms. Ice, NSAIDs, and rest are most helpful. I found the use of a sacroiliac belt, one of which I have designed for SI injuries, works even better than any rib wrap I've encountered for help with rib injury. (**wolfsibelt.com**) A rib wrap can help reduce discomfort. This belt also limits motion, which can alleviate some pain and protect from moving into a range of motion that can cause re-injury.

LUMBAR SPINE PROBLEMS

The lumbar spine is home to a lot of challenges regarding disease and injury. Because the lumbar spine is located at the bottom of the spinal column, it bears the most weight. The brick at the bottom of the building is more load bearing than the one at the top. Also, the lumbars lack collateral bone structures like the ribs in the thoracic spine. Just as the neck, the lumbar spine is more susceptible to injury in a flexed or rotated position. This part of the back has the same curve as the cervical spine. The lordotic curve of the lumbar spine is mechanically twelve times stronger than if the spine was straight. The straighter the spine the more physical load is placed on the bottom of the stack.

Injuries that are common to the lumbar spine include herniated and protruding discs, fractures, strains, sprains, and subluxations. Disease processes of the lumbar spine include degenerative disc disease, degenerative joint disease, facet syndrome, osteoporosis, pars defects, and stenosis, just to name a few. We are going to talk about the most common injuries suffered by training and how normal disease processes can complicate rehabilitation of these injuries. Lastly, we will discuss how to avoid back pain by checking your leg lengths after getting hip or knee replacement surgery.

A) Lumbar Strains and Sprains

Lumbar strains are very common in the low back. Usually, this is because we get into mechanically compromising positions. Sometimes, it's a challenge to consciously use our legs to lift heavy objects. Like the C-Spine (cervical spine), the lumbar spine is vulnerable to injury when in a flexed position. So, you will tend to hurt your back when bending over and lifting something heavy off the ground.

Keeping in mind this fundamental principle will help you prevent injuries at home or at the gym. Every time I see someone doing bent-over rows, I want to walk up to them and give them my business card. It's only a matter of time until they hurt themselves. There is no reason to put your spine into biomechanical compromise to exercise any muscles.

Even while in a neutral position, it's helpful to maintain this lumbar curve. It's useful to make sure you have good lumbar support when sitting at a desk for hours or driving a car, especially over long distances. Most people sit like the following picture on the left. Using a lumbar seat support can improve your posture tremendously as seen in the following picture on the right.

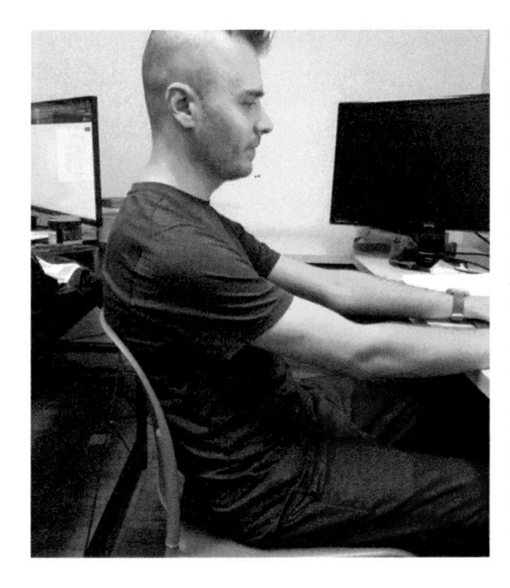

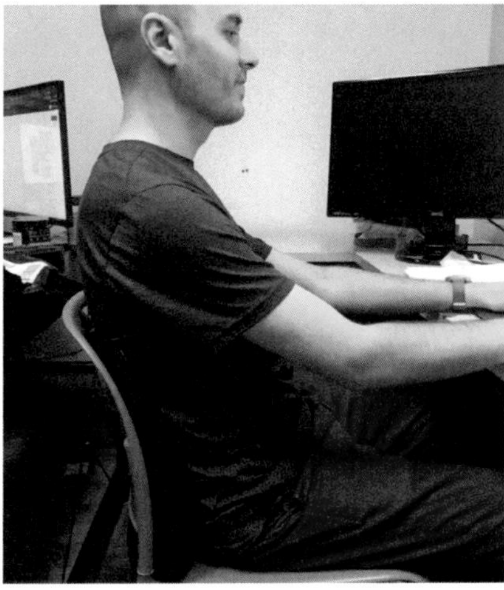

If your car seat or desk chair doesn't have good support, get a lumbar support from my website (**wolflumbarseat.com**) and simply put it behind your back. This lumbar support helps maintain your natural lumbar curve while sitting. This greatly decreases your likelihood of getting out of your seat with back pain.

Treatment of strains and sprains of the lumbar spine with the Big Five is quite effective.

B) Lumbar Misalignment (Subluxation) and Facet Syndromes

Bad mechanics, weak or strained ligaments, or trauma can cause a bone to misalign relative to another bone. Proper exercise technique is your best defense against knocking something out of whack in the gym. Maintain your lumbar curve while doing exercises. Avoiding certain toxic exercises like sit-ups, squats, deadlifts, and bent-over rows can help reduce the frequency of injury. Chapter 5, Section J discusses these routines in detail.

Reduction of misalignment by chiropractic treatment is the most effective. If there's a subluxation (misalignment), there is

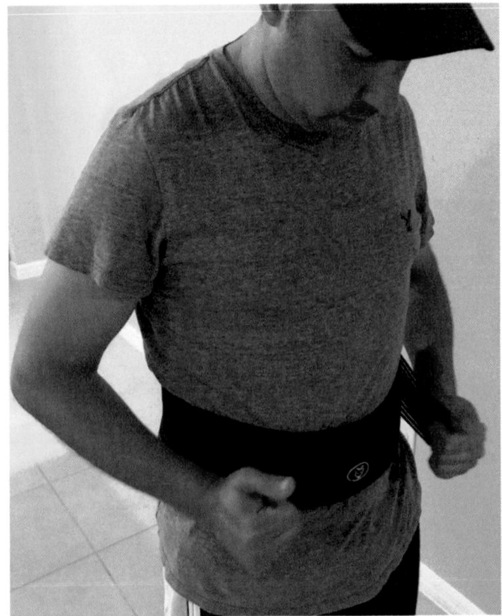

usually going to be a soft tissue strain component. For those issues, the Big Five treatment can help. When a strain to the low back occurs with this condition, it's helpful to brace the area in the acute phase(**wolflumbarbelt.com**).

Some facet syndromes are the direct result of arthropathy of the joint. This means the soft tissue lining of the joint has deteriorated to a degree and osteoarthritis has set in. The following x-rays demonstrate a normal spine and one with osteoarthritis.

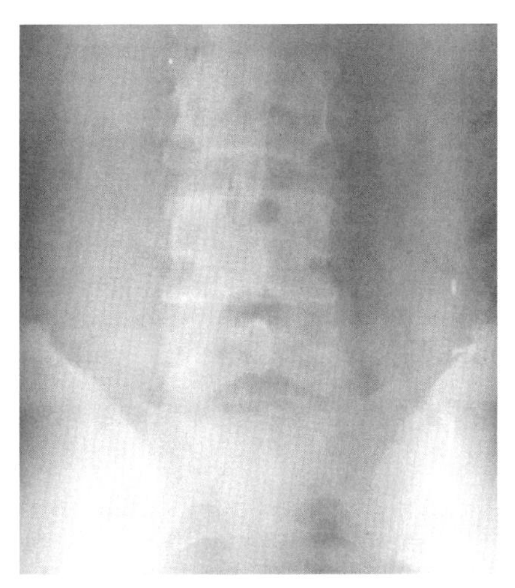

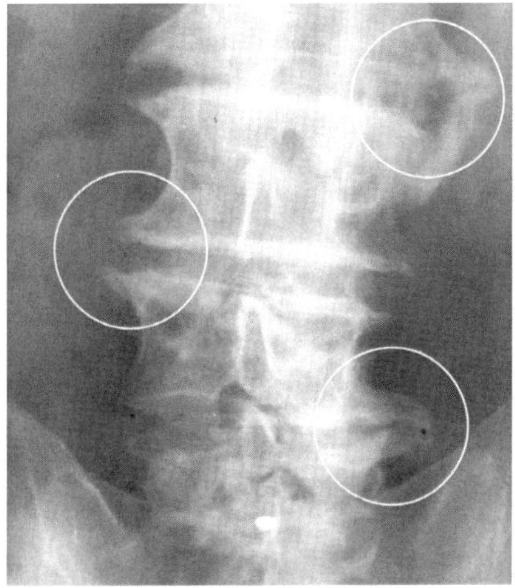

Sometimes short term prescription corticosteroids can help. Additionally, I've had some success referring patients for facet steroid injections to directly reduce the swelling. These methods can improve the quality of life with those that suffer from degenerative diseases. Using a lumbar brace while at work or while lifting weights at the gym can reduce injury by limiting the range of motion of the lumbar joints. The use of lumbar support belts helps reduce the chance of entering into a motion that compromises the degenerative joint (**wolflumbarbelt.com**).

C) Pars Defects

The pars interarticularis bone is a bone in the spine that bridges the upper and lower parts of the vertebrae. A pars defect is a fracture of this bone. Another name for this condition is spondylosis. Some textbooks say it's a congenital anomaly, but most doctors agree its etiology is from trauma at a very young age. The problem with pars defects is that the vertebrae starts to slide away from the corresponding vertebrae above.

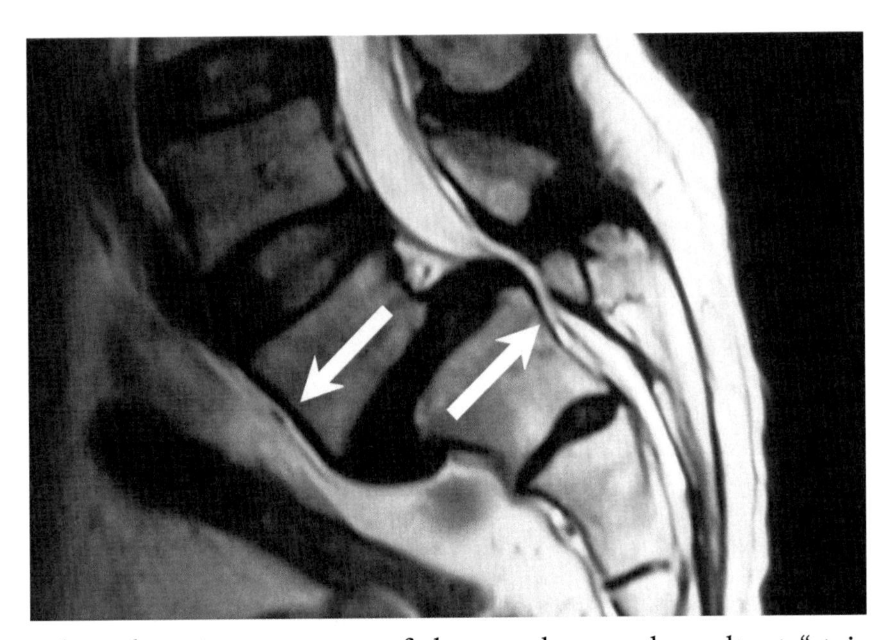

When there is movement of the vertebrae and resultant "stair stepping," this is called spondylolisthesis. This stair stepping presents some mechanic challenges when our body is put into flexion. There is no bony support holding the bones from slipping forward. As a result, there is extra stress placed on the soft tissue posterior elements of the spine. This predisposes the individual to the likelihood of more strains and sprains while in flexion. Not to mention, the more the vertebrae move forward, the more compromise to the spinal canal.

Patients with pars defects are very functional. Since these patients are more predisposed to soft tissue injury while in flexion, it's extremely important for these patients not to do exercises in flexion; for example, bent-over rows or deadlifts. The same treatment holds true as it does for any back strain. The Big Five is a great way of treating the acute phase. Maintaining a good lumbar curve is important too. Some stretching routines can help reduce pain and increase flexibility. Sleeping on your back is helpful, while sleeping on your stomach will exacerbate this condition. When a strain to the low back occurs with this condition, it's helpful to brace the area to avoid translation when bending forward. (**wolflumbarbelt.com**) Lastly, strengthening your core muscles helps stabilize this condition. The stronger and leaner your abdomen, the less pressure created making the spondylolisthesis worse. Patients with a large beer belly will suffer more with this condition than those with a flat stomach.

D) Lumbar Disc Protrusions and Herniations

Lumbar disc protrusions and herniations are a source of pain with many of us. The connective tissue in our spine degrades as we age, which can result in tears in the disc. Training with this injury can be dicey. In the cervical disc injury section of this chapter, we discussed the anatomy of the disc. Knowing this anatomy helps us understand the difference between a disc protrusion and a disc herniation.

There are a lot of names for these conditions. You might have heard of a slipped disc, disc bulge, disc desiccation, extruded disc, disc herniation, and ruptured disc. I think some of the literature is ambiguous when using these terms. So, let me lay it out for you as simply as I can. Let's throw "slipped disc" out the window. There's nothing slippery about a disc and this term draws no parallels. Only discs that dehydrate and lose water are prone to protrusions or herniations. Degenerative discs are always the ones that create problems. I think the terms bulge and protrusion are synonymous. Those names accurately represent what happens. When there is a tear in the outside layer (annulus) of the disc, the outward pressure exerted from the nucleus of the disc instigates a bulge or protrusion.

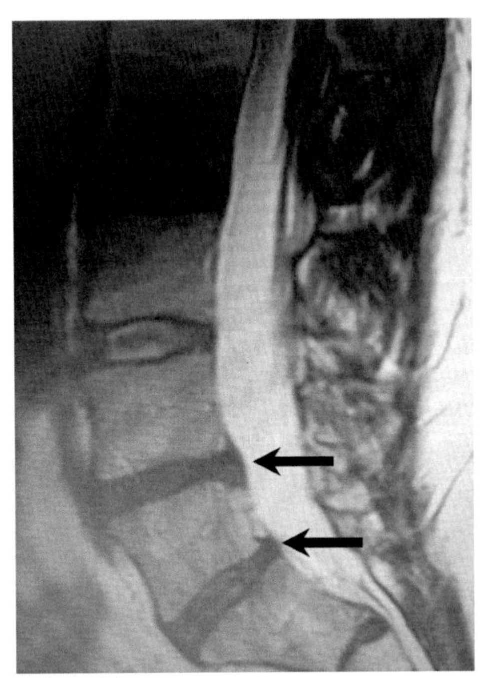

If the annulus has a large tear with enough outward pressure to extrude material from the disc's nucleus beyond its normal boundary or confines, this truly is a herniation.

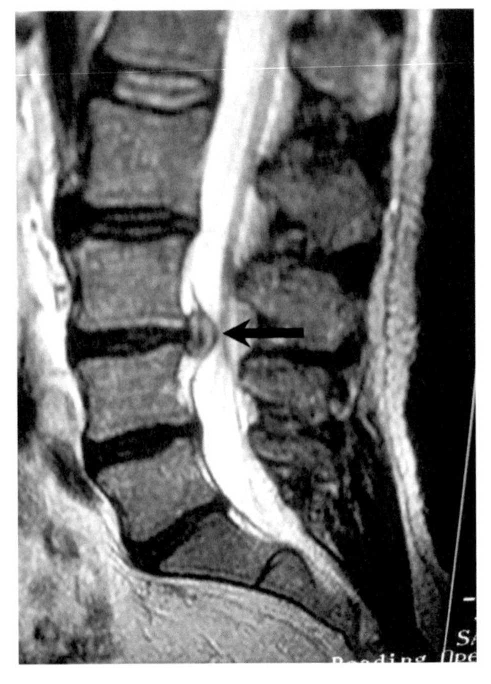

The amount of pain a lumbar disc injury provides depends on many factors. The size and shape of the canal can dictate the severity of pain. For example, a man with a small diameter spinal canal can suffer extreme pain from a small disc bulge. Conversely, a man with a huge herniation and an extremely large spinal canal can be almost asymptomatic. Remember, space is of the essence when it comes to the spinal cord. Anything that takes up space creates problems. Other tissue that could take up space could include cysts, facet joint enlargement, enlargement of the ligaments, or arthritic changes in the body of the vertebrae itself. The point here is that every case is unique and there are dozens of factors that determine the pain's type, severity, and duration. Instead of writing the next volume of War and Peace, we're going to focus on some basics that can give you the knowledge to seek out the care that you might need and determine how and when you can train with this injury.

Lumbar discs bear the most weight in a sitting position. Almost all spine problems are better when you sit. If you have pain in the low back and/or pain in the leg that is worse during sitting, odds are you have a hot disc. The sciatic nerve is the largest and longest nerve in the body and it's easy to test. In fact, the nerve is about the diameter of a pencil. The way to test this nerve is to sit in a chair and have someone lift each of your legs, one at a time. If this reproduces pain in your back, chances are you have a disc protrusion. If this test produces pain down your leg, chances are you have a disc herniation.

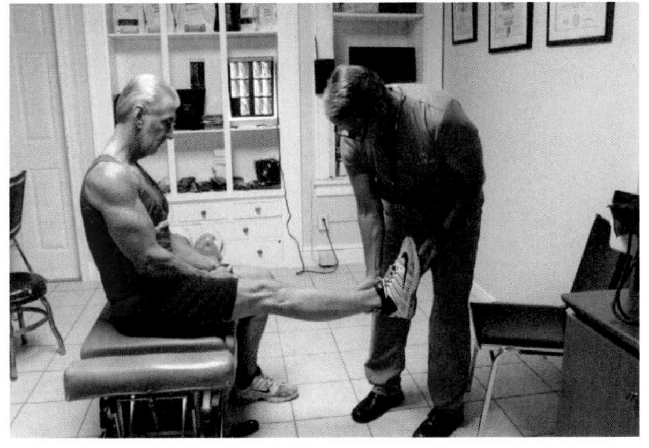

We can still function and even train with a disc protrusion. However, a disc herniation is a more difficult situation. If the nuclear material is extruded outside of its normal confines, trying to get that material to go back in through therapy is like trying to get toothpaste back in the tube. An MRI can determine a full blown herniation and the likelihood of surgical intervention. The size of the spinal canal can determine the severity of the condition. For example, if you have a small diameter canal, even a small disc bulge can cause a lot of pain and neurologic consequences. I have had patients that have had both a large diameter canal and a large herniation that were able to avoid the knife. The following MRI represents a large canal with three small disc protrusions that have little impact on the patient's quality of life.

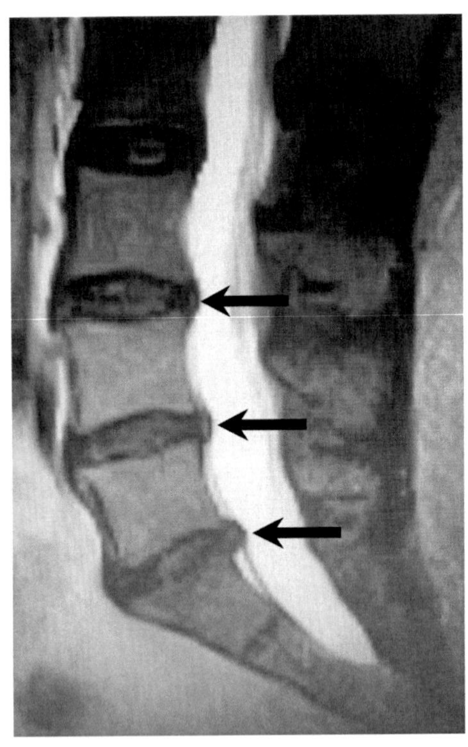

If this situation happens, the disc over time does resorb or shrink. Managing the swelling is the key with this one.

Motor function is the gold standard of neurosurgery. If the patient's motor skills are intact, surgery is not needed. Pain is not an indication for surgery. Let's give you a little neuroanatomy lesson. There are two networks of nerves that control the leg. Each of these networks are called a nerve plexus. First, we have the lumbar plexus. These nerves are from the first through the fourth lumbar nerves. Then we have the sacral plexus. These nerves develop from the fourth lumbar spinal nerve to the fourth sacral nerve. Basically, the lumbar plexus controls the sensory and motor function of the upper leg and rear end. The sacral plexus nerves control the rest of the leg.

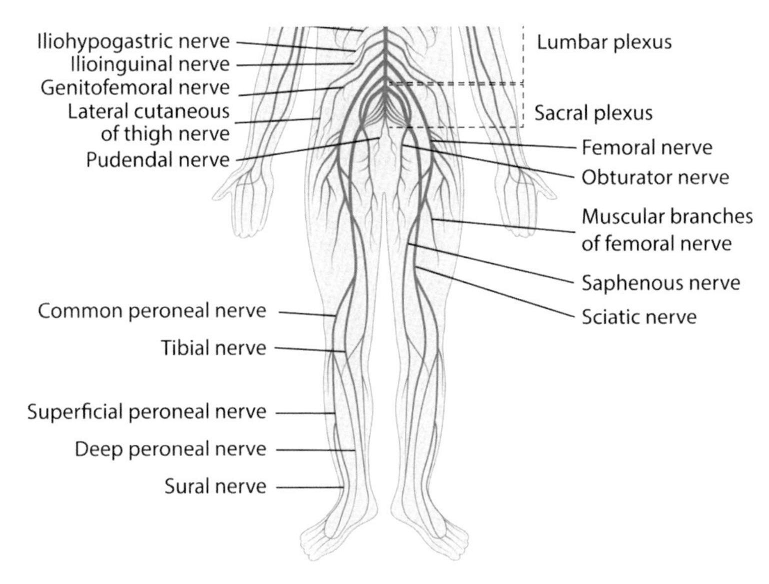

We are going to concern ourselves with the big three problem areas. Basically, because all of the weight is on the bottom of the stack, most lumbar disc problems arise from the bottom three segments. So, let's just focus on these. There are three main wires that go down the leg. The L4, L5, and S1 nerves. If the nerve function of these three nerves is good, there is no need for surgery. You might ask, how do we test these nerves? Here's how. The L4 nerve controls dorsiflexion of your foot. If you can stand on your heels, your L4 nerve is working just fine.

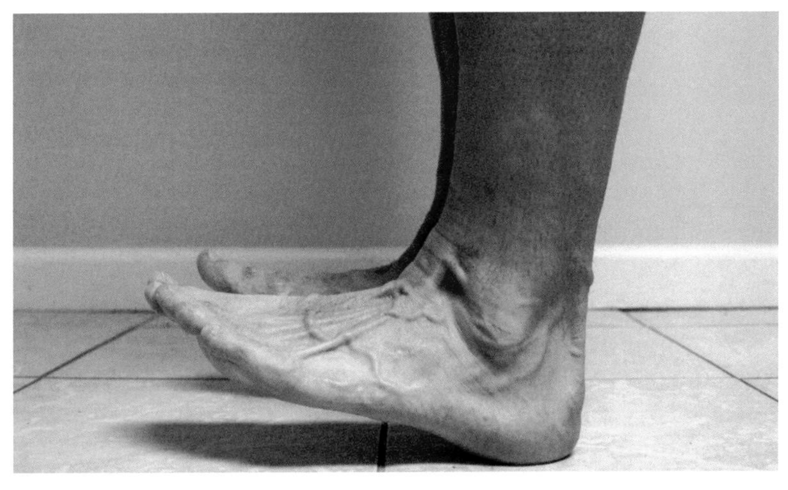

The L5 nerve uniquely controls the extension of your big toe. If you can wiggle your big toe, chances are the L5 nerve is working perfectly.

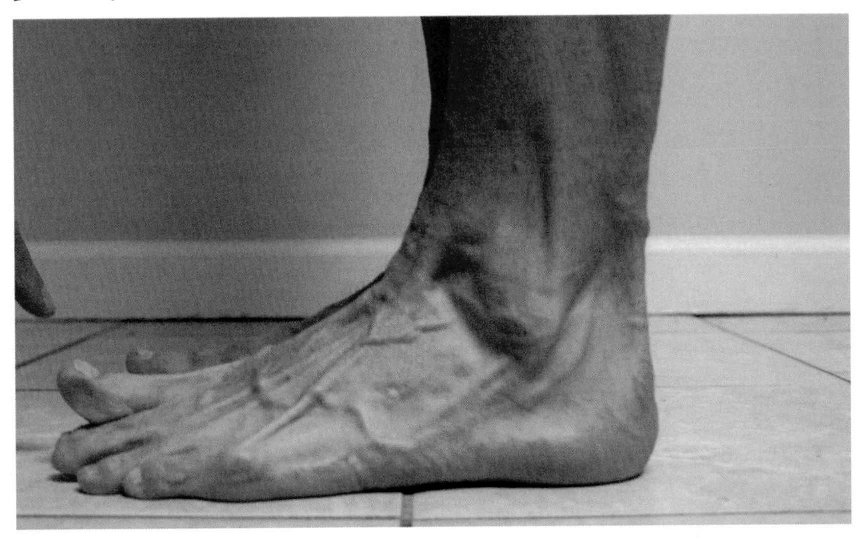

Lastly, the S1 nerve root controls plantar flexion of your foot. If you can stand on your tiptoes without a problem, this nerve is good to go, too.

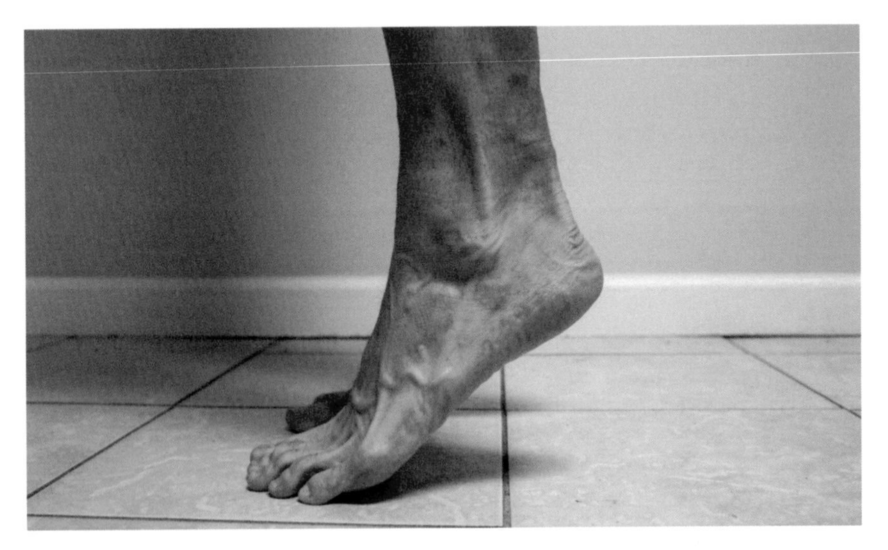

If you have lost any motor function with these nerves or any others, this is a medical emergency. Patients with lost function must decompress whatever is causing the pressure on the nerve immediately. If the nerve pressure is not relieved, permanent damage to the nerve and the structure it controls can take place. Do not take chances with nerve compression. If there is any doubt about loss of motor function, contact your chiropractor or medical doctor right away to be evaluated.

More than not, I have found that patients with lumbar disc issues get some warning signs from your body. So, the best treatment is not allowing it to happen at all. If you have progressing back discomfort, listen to your body and take it easy for a few weeks.

If you have a disc protrusion and you haven't lost any motor function, resting and treating with the Big Five is your best road to recovery. Clinically, I have found the short term use of corticosteroids very helpful in getting the patient out of the acute swelling phase of this injury. Flexion distraction is a form of a traction technique performed by a lot of chiropractors. This technique really works. So, if you're in the hot phase of a disc injury, seek out a chiropractor or physical therapist that performs this therapy.

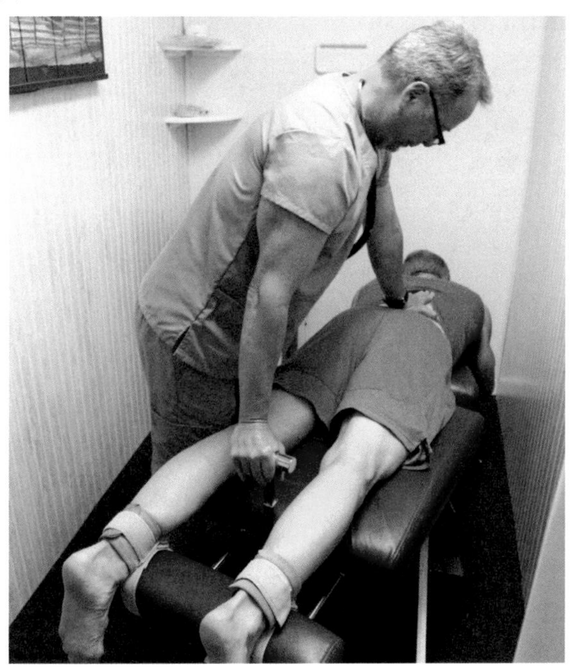

If treating this condition with these methods fails, I would recommend a consultation with an anesthesiologist for possible epidural steroid injections.

Training at the gym with a lumbar disc protrusion must be done with care. Exercises with a conscious effort to maintain proper posture must be a priority. Any exercise that puts your spine in flexion should be avoided. Because the disc bears the most weight while sitting, it's best to stay out of chairs as much as possible. The biggest issue I see with my disc patients is re-injury. Just as we're about to recover, the patient lifts groceries out of the trunk of the car or something similar, and we are back to square one – so be careful with this injury.

E) Lumbar Stenosis

Lumbar stenosis is my least favorite lumbar condition to treat. Most patients don't acquire this until after 60 or 70 years of age. Lumbar Stenosis is the narrowing of the spinal canal. There are several different mechanisms that cause this. Most commonly, it's from osteoarthritis.

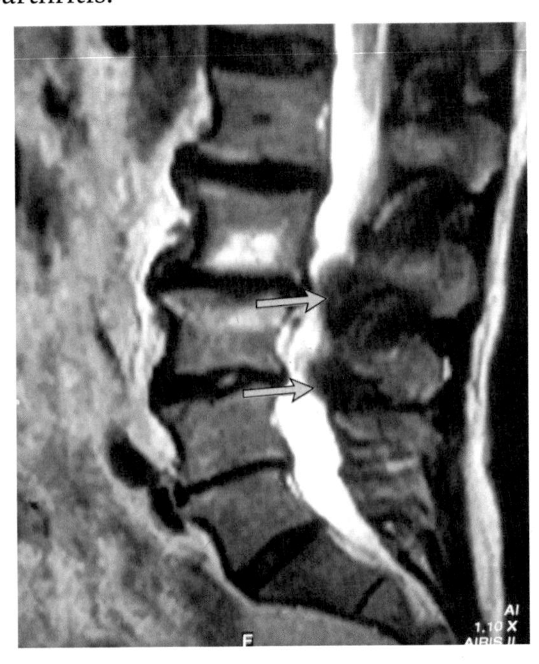

It can be from enlargement of one or more of the ligaments that run along the spine or around the facet joints. This enlargement is called hypertrophy. Ligament hypertrophy naturally occurs as we age. Other reasons include herniated discs, trauma, tumors, and diseases of the bones of the spine. Stenosis can occur in the actual spinal canal or the lateral recess where the peripheral nerves exit the spine. The previous MRI shows how arthritis can influence the diameter of the spinal canal and cause stenosis.

The symptoms of stenosis are similar to that of other spinal cord compression injuries. There could be numbness or tingling of the extremities. Weakness and fatigue occur frequently. The patient usually complains that if he walks for a period he notices his legs get achy, numb, and tired. As soon as the stenosis patient sits, the pain goes away.

Stenosis presents difficult challenges with training. Treatment with the Big Five can alleviate symptoms. Corticosteroid pills and steroid injections can buy you some time. When working out in the gym, you will have to employ rest periods, especially when doing cardio.

If the stenosis is severe enough to cause motor function loss, surgical intervention is needed immediately. Unfortunately, this condition will not get better on its own. Lumbar stenosis continues to progress. Therefore, if you are healthy enough to get the surgical procedure and your condition is significantly affecting your lifestyle, you should do so without delay. I have seen many patients put off the surgery only to have the condition worsen, and by that time other health complications disqualified the patient from being able to proceed with a surgical correction.

F) Hip and Knee Replacements

Yes, that's right. Hip and knee replacements are a leading cause of lumbar back problems. This is another sensitive subject for most chiropractors. When a prosthetic part is put in your body, it's usually because degeneration of that joint has occurred over time. Clinically, the problem is this: if there's degeneration on one side, there's probably degeneration on the other side. When these new parts are put in, the spacing between the bones is like brand new – at least for the side with the new prosthetic. The other joint is now responsible for the development of a shorter leg because of the decreased space from natural degeneration. For the life of me, I can't figure out why some orthopedic surgeons wouldn't check for leg length discrepancy after performing replacement surgery. A leg length difference accounts for pelvic tilt, which in turn results in lumbar misalignment. Clinically, I will see at least one patient a day that received a new hip or knee and now has back pain because of a leg length discrepancy. Simply putting a heel lift in the shoe on the short leg side will solve this problem quite nicely. (**wolfheellift.com**) If you have had a hip or knee replacement, you should have your chiropractor or physical therapist check for a leg length discrepancy. Let me show you an easy way to check your leg lengths.

Lay on your back, bend your knees and have someone move your knees from side to side as shown in the pictures below.

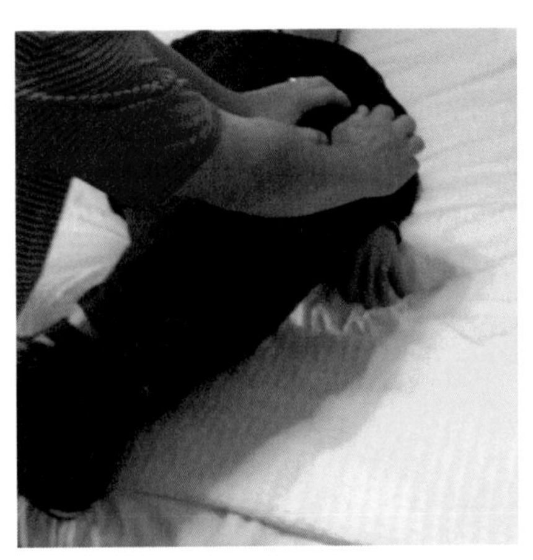

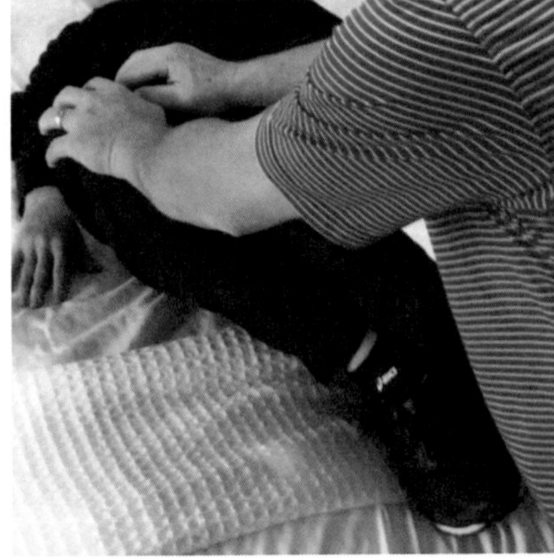

Then move the legs straight and look down at the heels as shown. Anyone can do it.

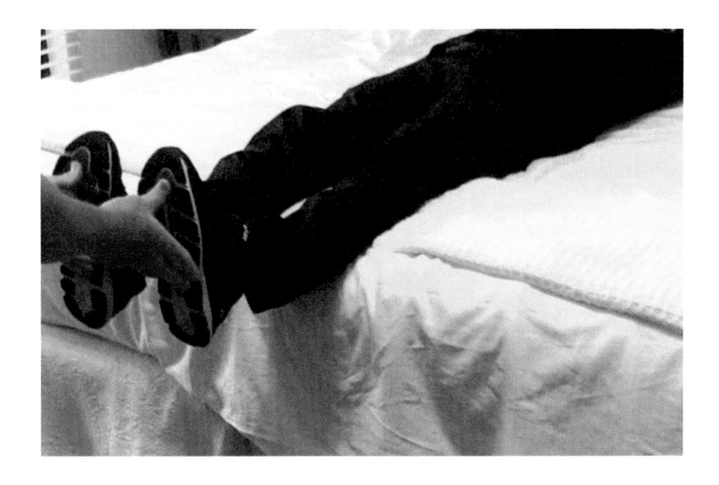

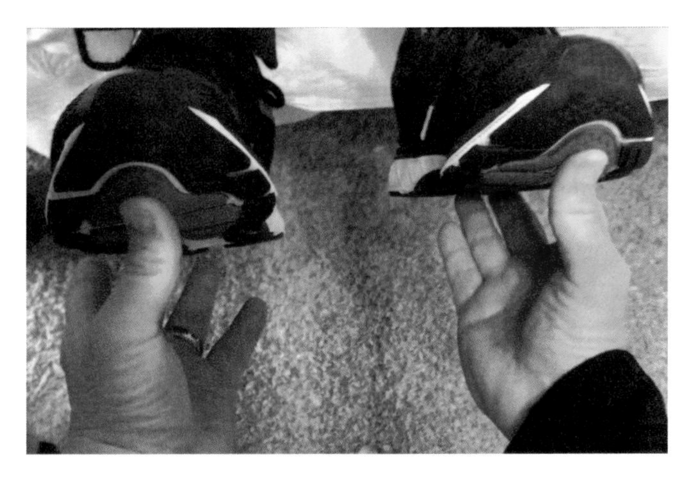

CHAPTER NINE

Extremity Injury, Prevention and Treatment

In this chapter, we will review common non-spinal injuries – the symptoms, causes, treatments, and preventative measures. We covered the foot in Chapter 3 and the spine in Chapter 8. This chapter will tackle extremity injuries that cause problems to all of us as we age. We will briefly cover important injuries absent Nuts and Bolts, as we did in the last chapter. Like Chapter 8, use this as a reference guide. If you don't have a specified injury, just skip ahead until there's one of interest to you. If you're active, you probably will encounter one or more of these at one time or another. We will start from the bottom of the body and work our way up.

In the last chapter, I coined the phrase "Big Five" for the five most common ways to treat soft tissue injuries, whether it be the spine or in the extremities. If you skipped over that section in the very beginning of the chapter, you might want to page back and glance over it because the material is useful in discussing ways of treating soft tissue injury.

ANKLE STRAINS AND SPRAINS

The terms"strain"and"sprain"are sometimes use interchangebly. However, they are not exactly the same. Technically speaking, a strain is an injury to the tendon and muscle tissue. A sprain is an injury to the ligament. Ligaments have less blood flow than tendons and muscles, so sprains take longer to heal.

The Big Five is definitely the way to go in treating either of these injuries. When it comes to the ankle, the acute phase of injury is a good time to stabilize the ankle with athletic tape and/or ankle support. The following picture shows an ankle x-wrap that works the best to allow both flexibility and support. (**wolfanklesleeve.com**).

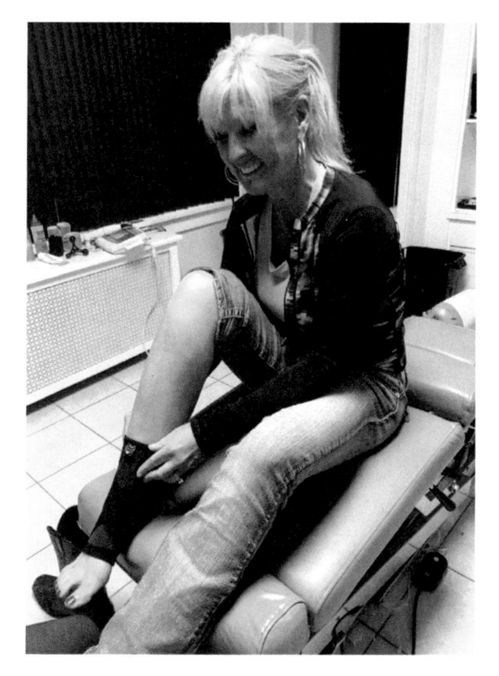

If you have chronic ankle sprains, chances are you have a biomechanical weakness or instability. This can be caused by either the ligament or tendon being stretched to a point where it's lost its resilience. When this occurs, ankle supports and taping do a good job of picking up the slack for these compromised tissues.

Another possible mechanical issue could be an anatomical short leg. The short leg side is where the ankle will sprain or strain most of the time. I can't tell you how many thousand times I've looked down at a patient lying on my table and saw the following:

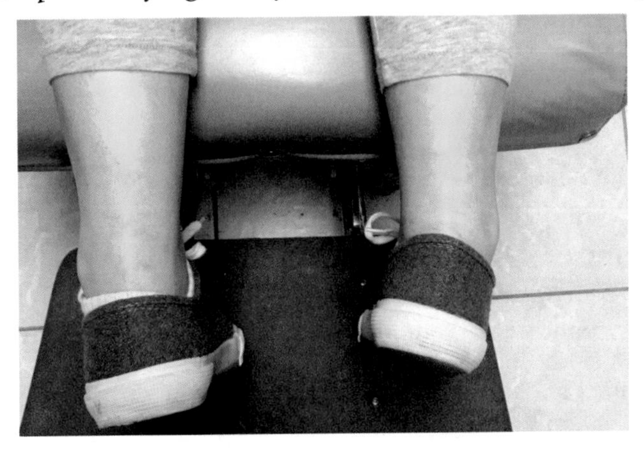

You can clearly see by the picture that the short leg is the one that's been repeatedly sprained over the years. Because of this, you can see a plastic deformity of the lateral structures, resulting in the foot being inverted. Also, the bottom of the shoe on the short side will show more wear-and-tear. Simply putting a heel lift in the shoe of the short leg side will eradicate this problem. (**wolfheellift.com**). Doing so will exponentially decrease the likelihood of continually spraining the ankle. An added benefit to putting the lift in the shoe is that it will help decrease the likelihood of other injuries up the kinetic chain.

The best way to determine if there's an anatomical short leg is to get X-rays taken while in a standing position. These weight-bearing views will demonstrate any leg length discrepancy and show mechanical compensations that can occur in the knee or spine. Most doctors don't order weight-bearing X-rays for their patients, which is a blunder on the part of the medical profession. Most imaging centers and hospitals take spine and hip X-rays while the patient is lying down because it's easier and quicker when trying to position the patient. At the very end of Chapter 8 we have pictures demonstrating a simple way of checking leg lengths. Also, you can view a video on **DrDeanWolf.com** to see how to check for leg length discrepancies.

Training with a strain or sprain of the ankle can be done if stability is restored. Of course, I wouldn't recommend mountain climbing if you're in the acute phase of injury. Rest, the Big Five, taping, and bracing go a long way with this injury. If you have ankle swelling and pain without trauma, it's important to see a healthcare professional for blood work to rule out gout or a vascular or cardiac problem.

Knee Disorders

There are four ligaments and two pieces of cartilage that make up the knee compartment. Outside of the knee, there are a bunch of tendons that connect the quadriceps and hamstrings muscles. Also, there are three bones associated with this hinge joint we call the knee. Instead of going over every possible structural abnormality, I am going to focus on the most prevalent injuries and what we can do to manage them and how to train with them.

Issues that affect the knee include: osteoarthritis, chondromalacia patellae (patellofemoral syndrome), and tears of the anterior cruciate ligament (ACL), the posterior cruciate ligament (PCL), and the medial (MCL) and lateral collateral ligaments (LCL). Other common problems include cartilage tears of the medial and lateral meniscus, hamstrings, and quadriceps tendon, as well as tendinitis of the patellar tendon. Runners are known to suffer from iliotibial band syndrome. Lastly, there's the infamous total knee replacement. Let's take them one at a time.

A) Arthritis of the Knee

Osteoarthritis of the knee is common for people after 50 years of age. This inflammatory condition is the direct result of erosion of the cartilage of the knee often caused by translation. Symptoms include joint pain, loss of motion, stiffness, and swelling. Diagnosis is made by X-ray.

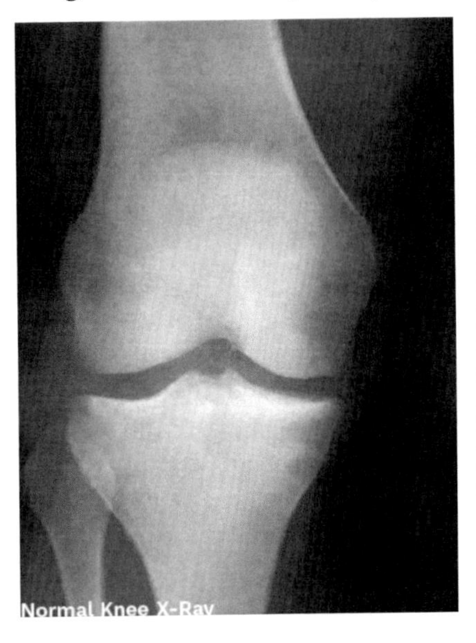

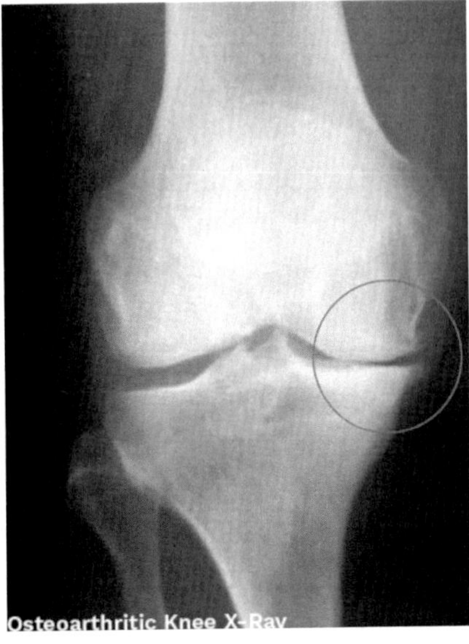

Here's an example of a condition where it makes sense to not be carrying around any extra weight. The process of arthritis may not necessarily be reversed but symptoms can be managed with treatment using the Big Five. TENS units can provide a lot of relief with arthritic conditions. (**wolftensunit.com**) Supplementation with glucosamine (**wolfjointrebuild.com**) and Type II collagen are also very helpful. Orthotics (**wolforthotics.com**) can be the most helpful because they eliminate pronation of your foot. Decreased pronation will lessen the likelihood of shear-causing issues such as tibial rotation and varus force.

Bracing of the knee helps with stability, which can reduce pain. I like two braces for arthritic knee support and ample range of motion. A kneecap support brace helps stop the kneecap from moving. Kneecap movement can aggravate arthritis. (**wolfkneebrace.com**).

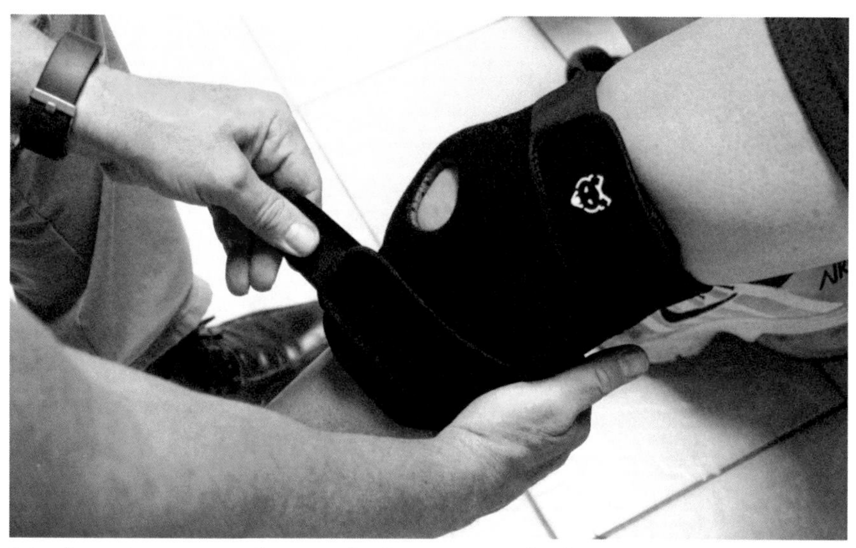

My favorite way to brace the knee is with the X Strap KneeWrap. This device gives excellent support while allowing maximum mobility and at the same time providing the most comfort.

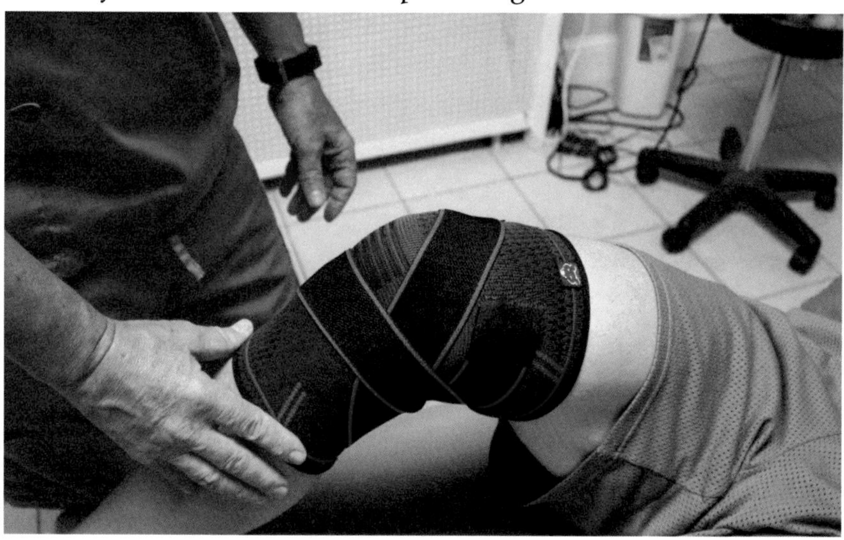

(**wolfkneesleeve.com**) If NSAIDs don't provide enough relief, prescription steroids can help. Steroid injections can buy you some time. When all else fails, knee replacement surgery might be indicated.

Osteoarthritis should not be an excuse to become sedentary.

You can and should train with osteoarthritis. Patients might note a decrease in pain with activity. This is because mechanical movement naturally disperses edema, which is the swelling that can occur from the accumulation of excess fluid in the joint. Be cautious during hamstring exercises, making sure not to approximate your heel to your leg to such a degree that you put a scissors-like shear into the back of your knee. I would be careful and eliminate deep knee bends or any other motion that bends the knee excessively. Our bodies are wonderfully wired with sensory nerves, so listen to your body and let pain be your guide. Never exercise a joint into pain.

B) Chondromalacia Patellae and Patellofemoral Syndrome (PFS)

While these two conditions are separate problems, they have similar causation and identical fixes. Chondromalacia patellae is a condition of the wearing down of cartilage under the kneecap. This is so common for 50 year-olds that people in this age group are more likely to have it than not. Patellofemoral syndrome, also known as runner's knee or jumper's knee, is an affliction found in many young athletes that do a lot of running and jumping.

First, we have to understand how the kneecap works. The patella (kneecap) is in your body to act as a pulley to help with the mechanical advantage of the quadriceps tendons. I've read textbooks which explain that the kneecap acts as a shield to the knee. If that were true, we would have an elbow cap. Because of the increased force needed to create leg extension by the strongest muscles in our body, the kneecap acts like a pulley system to aid in helping us get off the ground or out of a chair. The kneecap basically floats in front of our knee. The four strong quadriceps tendons that go over and around the structure of the kneecap and insert into the lower leg play a role in the position of the kneecap. Underneath the kneecap is a little groove in the femur bone called the trochlear groove. The shape of the kneecap reminds me of a teardrop diamond. The top is dome shaped, and the side underneath comes to a point. The point of the diamond fits in the groove of the femur. The shape of the bones and the associated muscle and tendon structures hold the kneecap in place. The following X-ray represents the normal position of the kneecap of a 20 year-old person.

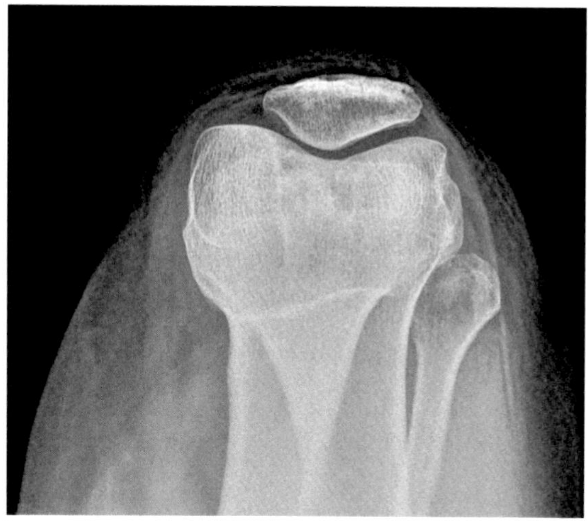

Both chondromalacia patellae and patellofemoral syndrome are manifestations of the same mechanics with different outcomes. In both of these conditions, the lateral quadriceps muscles become so much stronger than the medial quadriceps muscle for different reasons. In the case of chondromalacia patellae, it is from disuse. As we age, we don't bend our knees to pick something off the ground as much as a young person does. Look at the following picture on the left of how a 20 year-old man picks up a pencil off the floor versus how a 50 year-old man does the same in the picture on the right.

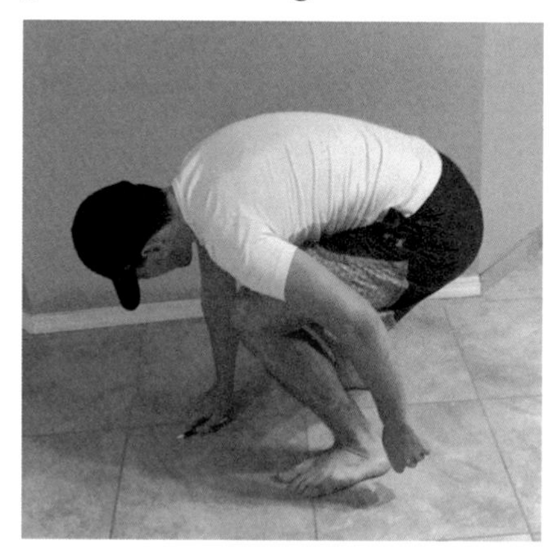

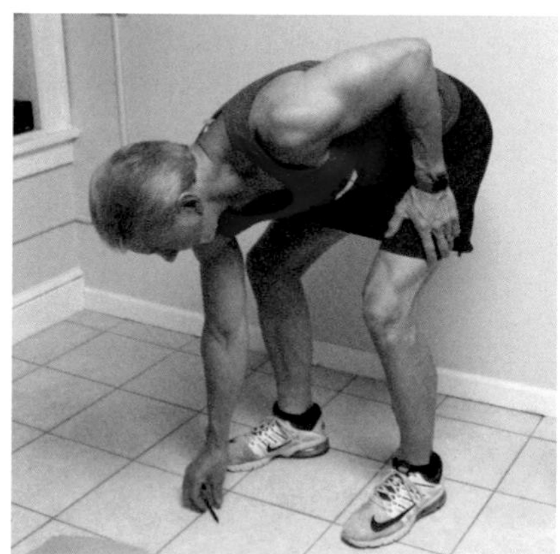

Can you see the difference in knee bend? As a result, the outside quads become stronger over time, relative to the inside quads. In the case of patellofemoral syndrome (PFS), the exact same thing happens to young athletes for an obvious reason: they are exercising the outside quads way more than the inside quad. This is why imbalance occurs. For example, a basketball player runs up and down the court for miles during a game. All the while running and jumping, rarely do they get into an athletic position similar to a catcher in baseball, so they never work their inside quadricep.

When suffering chondromalacia patellae, the underside of the kneecap rubs against the femoral condyles because it's pulling to the strong side. Look at the following X-ray of a person in his 50s.

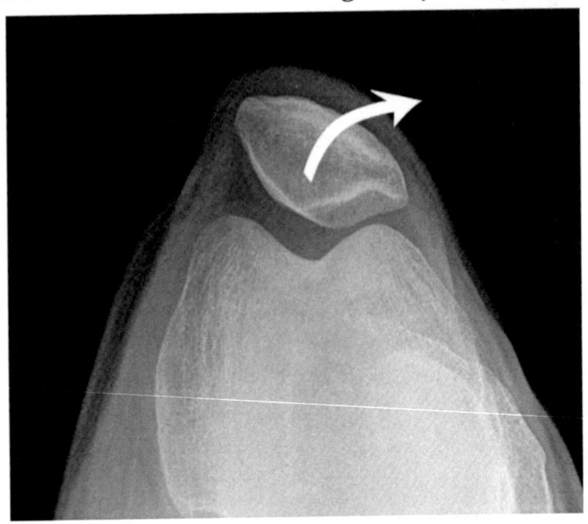

Notice how, in comparison to the X-ray of the person in their twenties, the kneecap isn't sitting in the groove? In this case, the bone sitting off to the side rubs against the other bone. This constant, year-after-year grinding starts to erode the cartilage and create pain and inflammation. The same thing happens in young athletes with PFS.

Treatment in both of these conditions includes strengthening of the medial quad muscles. Leg extension machines achieve this the best. During leg extensions, the vastus medialis – the muscle in the quadriceps that extends the knee – is isolated quite nicely.

Another very effective way to manage this condition is with a cho strap, sometimes called a "jumper's knee strap." (**wolfkneestrap.com**).

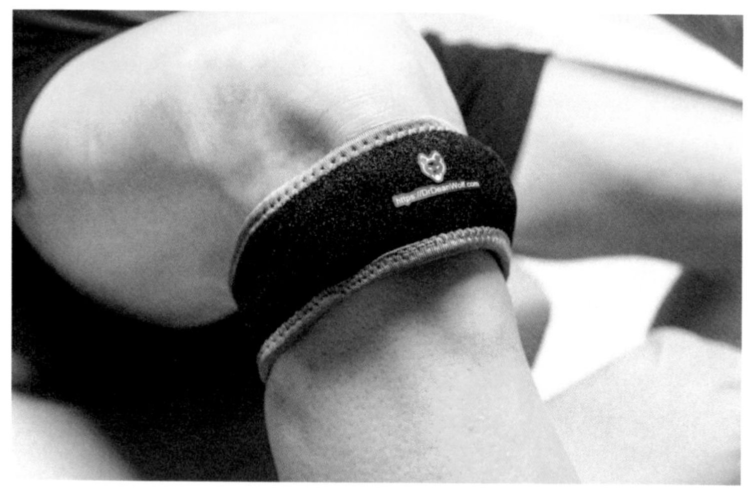

The first time I saw this strap, I thought to myself, "This little thing isn't going to do anything." I couldn't have been more wrong. The simple downward pressure helps the kneecap glide in its natural groove and the pressure on the patellar tendon reduces pain (**wolfdualknee.com**). I've even recommended the strap for patellar tendinitis. This condition presents itself with pain above the kneecap. Some individuals prefer the dual strap that puts pressure above as well as below the knee.

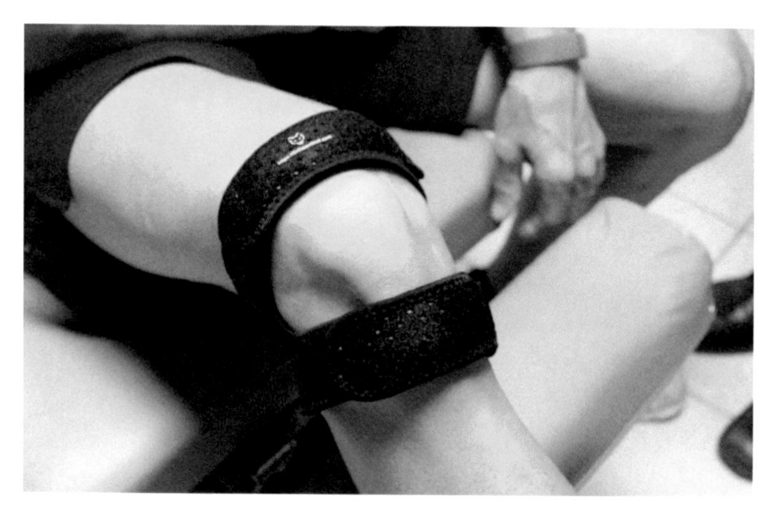

C) Ligament Sprains and Tears of the Knee

As you may remember from Chapter 4, the knee is made up of four ligaments. Two of them are the anterior cruciate (ACL) and posterior cruciate (PCL), which limit front and back translation of the knee. There are also the medial collateral ligament (MCL) and lateral collateral ligament (LCL). These other two ligaments help stabilize side to side motions of the knee.

Tears to any knee ligaments are quite serious. Usually, tears to this structure occur in younger athletes from trauma. In older patients, it's more a function of a translation deformity from normal degeneration that causes microtrauma over time. Often in trauma situations, more than one structure is torn. For example, a typical football knee injury will involve tears to the ACL, MCL, and medial meniscus.

Symptoms of a tear include a popping or snapping sound in the knee at the time of the tear. Usually, this is followed by extreme pain. Swelling persists immediately with an inability to fully straighten your knee. A doctor can detect a tear of the ACL by performing the Lachman's Test. The patient will lie on his back with the knee at an approximately 90° angle. Then the doctor will hold the femur with one hand and place the other hand on the back of the calf, pulling up and away from the knee. If there is movement or translation of the lower leg bone, you can be pretty sure there's a tear.

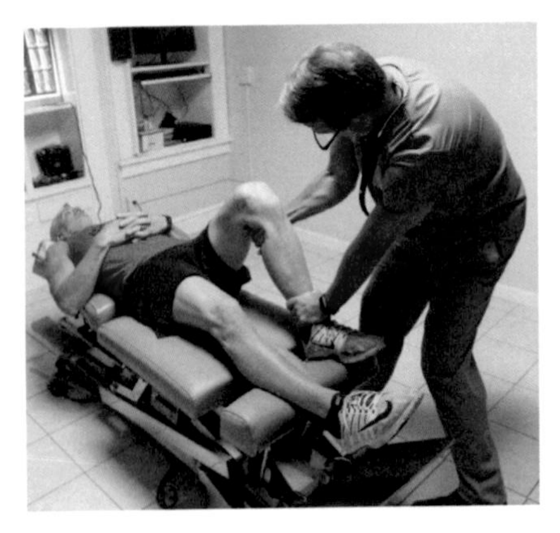

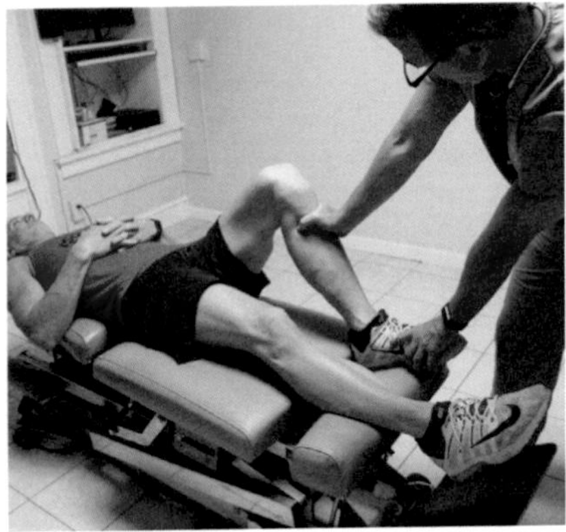

The reverse motion placed into the knee is performed to diagnose a PCL tear, as shown in the previous picture. The PCL ligament is much stronger than the ACL – if torn, there are usually multiple injuries of the knee to go along for the ride.

To diagnose an MCL tear, a patient will lie in a prone position (stomach facing down) while the doctor pushes with an inward force to look for looseness of the joint; alternatively, the doctor would push outward to determine if there is an LCL tear.

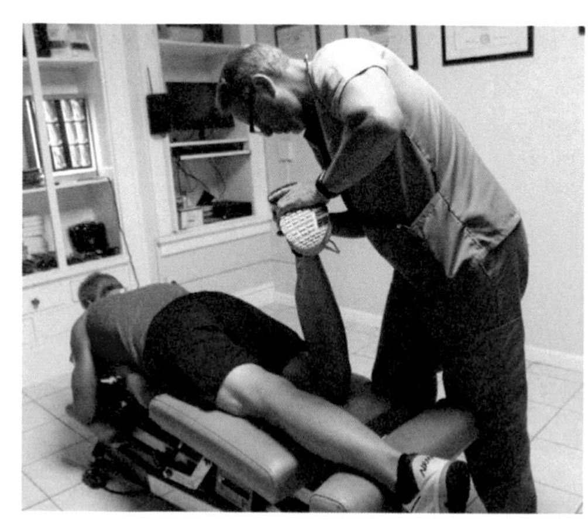

If there are sprains to these structures, rest is important. Anything to increase blood flow is useful, so the Big Five treatments are very helpful. After you are out of the acute sprain phase, your workouts should resume slowly. Let pain be your guide. If the pain is minimal, I'd recommend doing light sets to help with flexibility and blood flow. Quadriceps and hamstring exercises help with the knee's stability. As the discomfort diminishes, you can increase the weight.

Usually, when you stretch the ligament enough to create a sprain, there is going to be more laxity in the joint, thereby predisposing you to more injury. So, bracing and wrapping the knee during athletic activities help decrease the likelihood of re-injury. (**wolfkneebrace.com**)

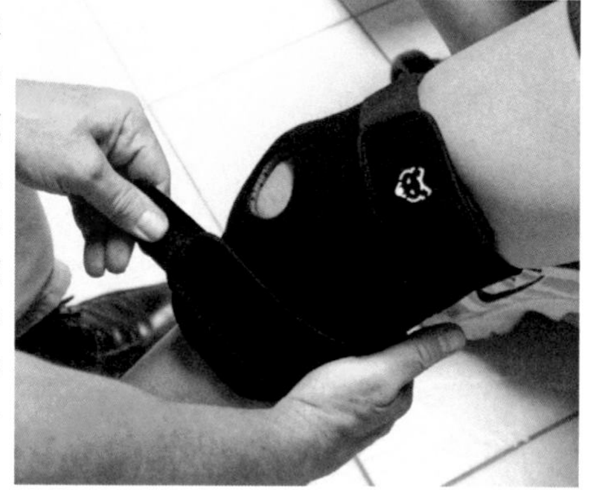

If there's a partial tear of the ACL, you can manage without surgery. If there's a complete tear to any knee ligament, surgery to reattach the ligament is necessary. When the ACL or PCL ligament tear, forward and backward movement over the cartilage predisposes the cartilage itself to injury. When the MCL and LCL tear, there is side-to-side shear force that can create a tear in the meniscal cartilage.

Strengthening the hamstrings can dramatically help ACL patients. Quad exercises help the PCL patient. Bracing the knee can help stabilize a partial tear. (**wolfhingedknee.com**) Bracing, coupled with strengthening routines, can keep you functional.

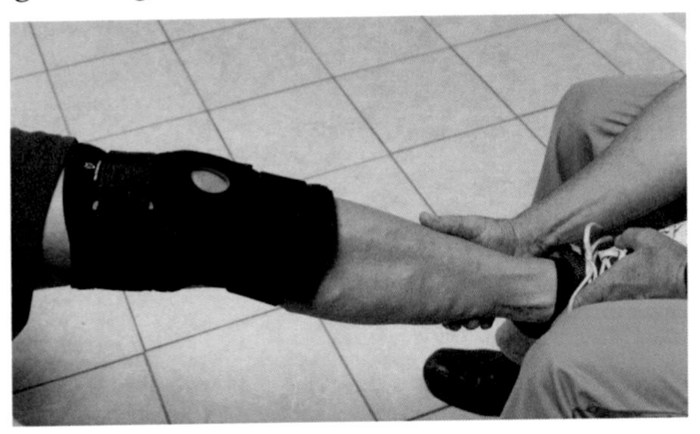

Once again, the Big Five treatments can manage symptoms, but this injury tends to be on the serious side. Therefore, I almost always recommend an orthopedic surgeon consultation.

D) Meniscal Strains and Tears

The knee is one of the largest joints in the body. The knee has two C shaped pieces of cartilage called the medial meniscus (MM) and the lateral meniscus (LM). Like most cartilage, the meniscus is vulnerable to torsion (twisting) forces. Pivot motions can get you in trouble.

As we age, the cartilage in the knee loses water and becomes brittle like other fibrocartilage in our body. Meniscal tears are more prevalent with age. At age fifty, twenty percent of all men have meniscal tears without symptoms. At 70 years old, 56% of all men have tears that don't hurt at all. With this in mind, it becomes apparent that arthroscopic surgery isn't always needed for meniscal tears. Most texts agree that the knee pain suffered in most patients is from the arthritic component. That said, acute onset tears of the meniscus can be extremely painful. Surgical intervention is quite helpful. On the other hand, the meniscus can heal on its own if the tear isn't too severe.

When training, it's important not to compromise the meniscus of the knee. Torsion forces, such as a twisting action to the knee, create the most mechanical problems. Additionally, it's mechanically problematic to get the knee in full flexion. Full flexion may occur in instances when there is a deep knee bend or bicycle riding with the seat in the lowest setting. Some posterior shear occurs in this position and is more likely to create a tear of the posterior horn of the meniscus. This scissor-like motion can occur in the back of the knee while riding a bike. Whether using an exercise bike or bicycle, it's important not to have the seat too low. The higher the seat, the less the knee bends at the top of the stroke cycle. When injured, using bracing helps reduce translation effects while exercising. (**wolfkneebrace.com**)

Another thing to watch with a weak knee is your leg length. Leg length discrepancies will account for chronic knee problems. Usually, the short leg side is the one with the bad knee. Simply putting a heel lift (**wolfheellift.com**) in the shoe on the short leg side can eliminate knee pain.

E) Muscle and Tendon Strains of the Knee

Muscle and tendon strains occur quite often in the active 40-plus body. There are a couple of common strains we will cover in this section. Patellar tendinitis and quadriceps tendinitis are the most common. Less commonly, you can get tendinitis in the hamstrings and calf muscles.

Using the Big Five treatments is best for tendinitis issues. I have found straps and braces to be excellent tools to help you continue to work out with less pain. Let's go over how to wrap or brace for each of these conditions.

1. Patellar tendinitis (jumper's knee) presents with pain just over the top of the kneecap or just below the kneecap. Wearing a cho strap (**wolfkneestrap.com**) above or below the knee can make a huge difference. This isn't a cure, but it sure helps reduce discomfort while working out. Some like the dual strap (**wolfdualknee.com**) if there's pain in both the top and bottom of the kneecap. The dual straps works best for those that suffer from severe kneecap hypermobility issues.

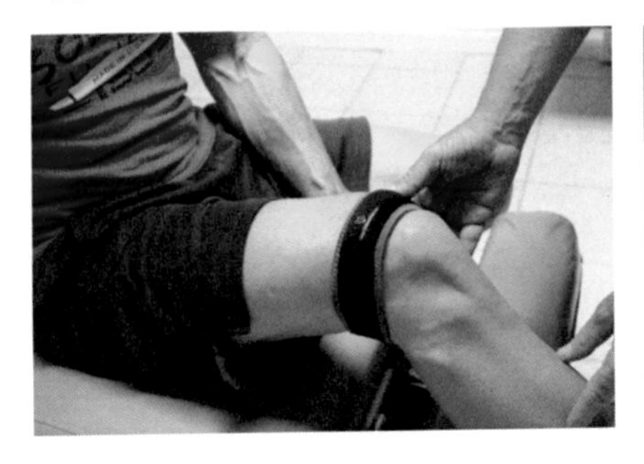

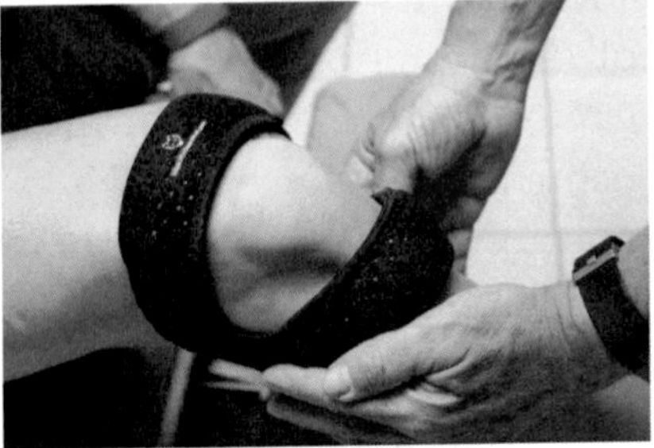

2. Quadriceps tendinitis can occur around the knee, too. In this case, I might turn the cho strap a little more to the affected side. The picture on the left shows how to apply the strap for medial quad tendinitis and the view on the right shows how to put the strap on with lateral quad tendinitis.

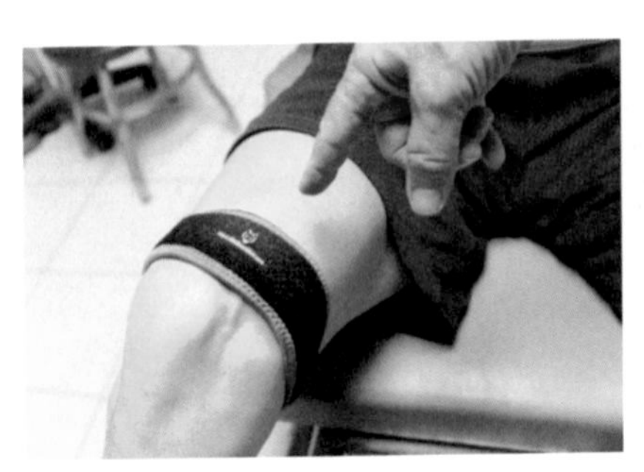

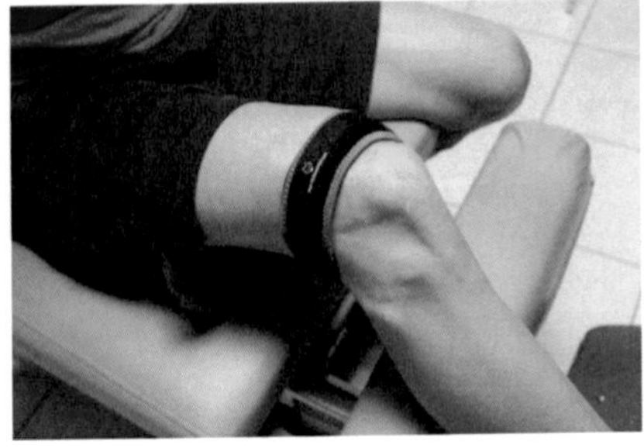

3. Quadriceps muscle strain can occur with stop-and-start sports, like racquetball or tennis. I hurt my quad muscle bowling several consecutive games during one tournament. The quad wrap works great to get you through the acute phase and enables you to keep playing. (**wolfthighwrap.com**)

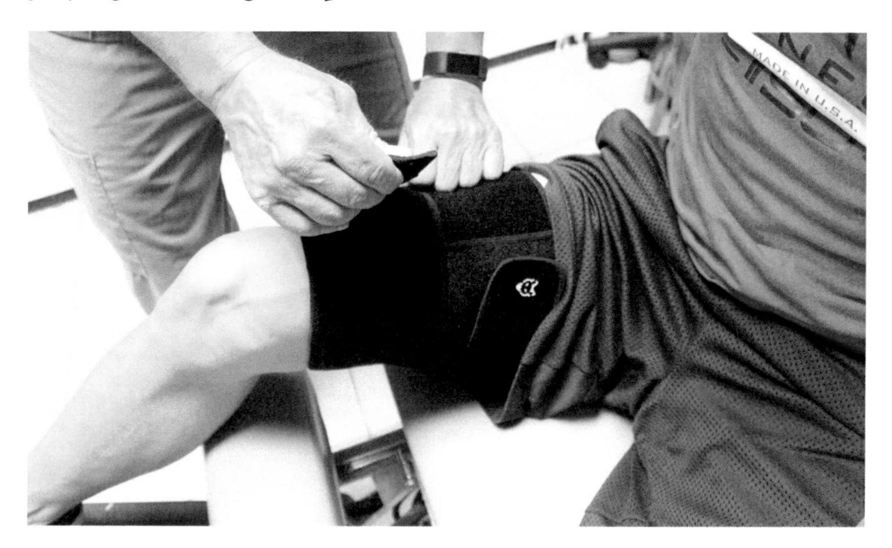

4. The biceps femoris muscles are known as the hamstrings. These are the muscles that make you run. If you want to run faster, strengthen your hamstrings. The stronger your hamstrings are the faster you will run. Hamstring strains are very common and usually occur with running-type injuries. Worse yet is a tear of one or both of the hamstrings. This usually occurs at the proximal (closest to the center of the body) part of the hamstrings. If there is a tear of the hamstring, you will hear an audible pop that is followed by moderate-to-severe pain. When this occurs, there will be bleeding under the skin. In about a day or two, your leg will look black-and-blue – something like the following picture.

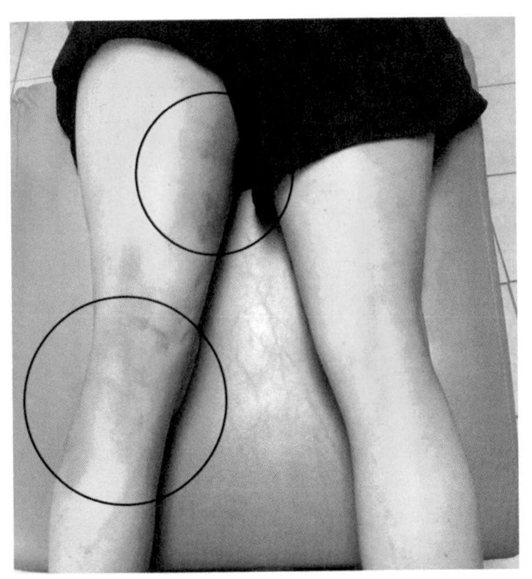

This is an example of a mild tear of the hamstrings. A quad wrap does wonders for relieving pain for this injury and getting you back on track.

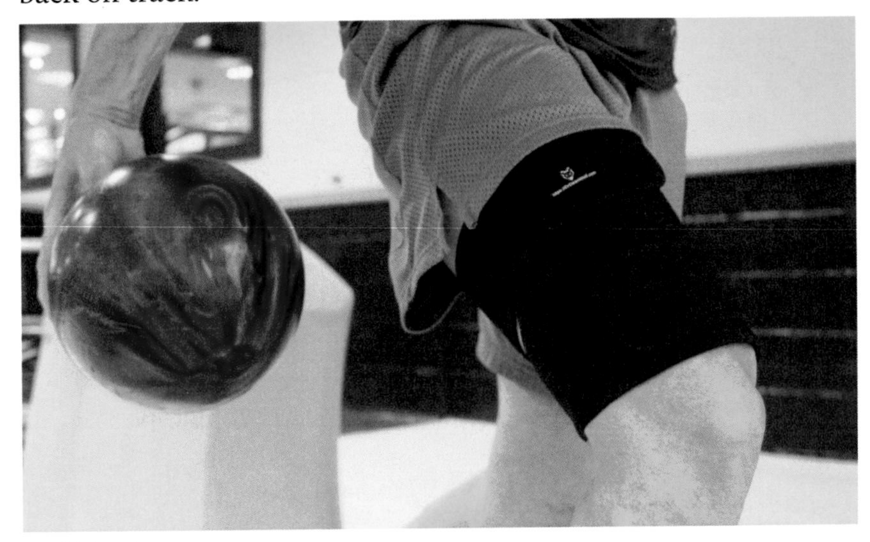

wolfthighwrap.com

If you have no palpable lumps, chances are that you haven't torn enough of the tendon or muscle to necessitate surgical intervention. However, if you find a large mass to be present anywhere on the leg, you must be evaluated right away by a chiropractor or orthopedist. The hamstrings (biceps femoris muscles) insertions can get tendinitis, too. When this has happened to a patient, I have used a cho strap on them with great success. Simply turn the strap around.

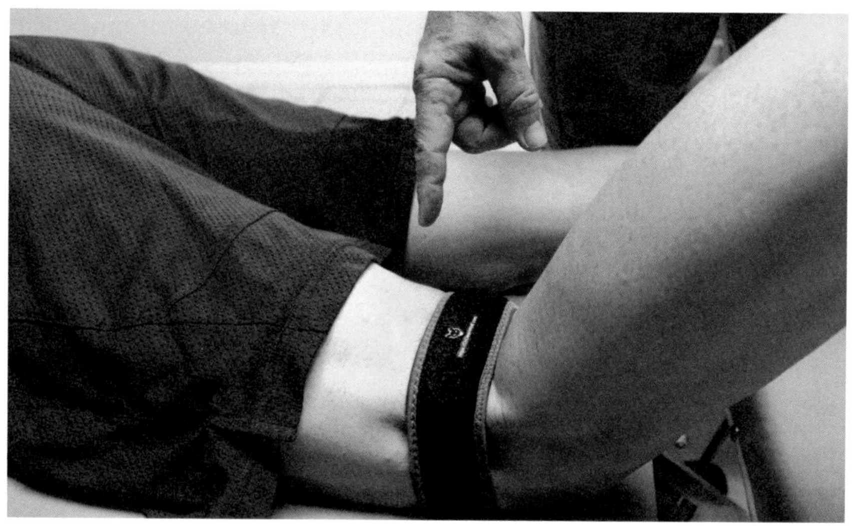

5. *The calf muscle (gastrocnemius) strain and tendinitis* are more difficult. Injury to this muscle can take a long time to recover from. The medial head of the calf is usually the one involved. A large compression wrap (**wolfcalfwrap.com**) is useful in helping you get around with this injury.

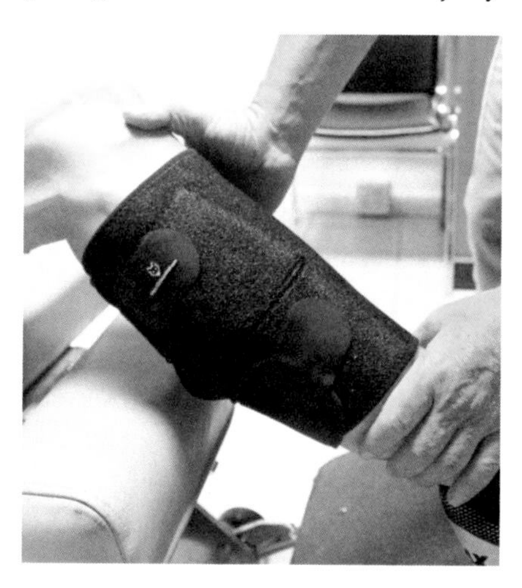

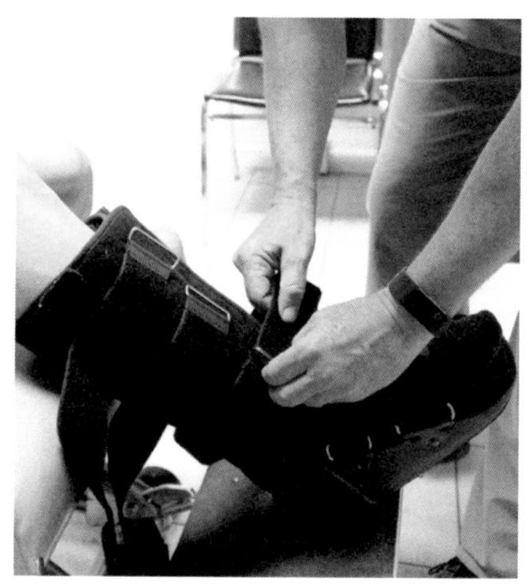

In severe cases, there could be a tear in the gastrocnemius muscle. If this is the case, it's important to completely immobilize this area by wearing a foot boot.

Hip and Pelvic Disorders

The pelvic area has a lot of large muscle attachments and therefore can be the home of many strains and sprains. Most strains of these muscles resolve quite nicely with the Big Five treatment and rest. Hip flexor strains, lumbopelvic strains, gluteal strains, and upper hamstrings and upper quadriceps strains are self-limiting and usually heal on their own. On the other hand, there are a few pelvic soft tissue injuries that could use a little help and respond well to a specific treatment. We will focus on these injuries in this section.

A) Pelvic Misalignment

Pelvic misalignment is probably the most commonly treated condition in a chiropractor's office and probably the single biggest oversight by the medical community. The pelvis is comprised of six bones that serve as the foundation of our spine. The strongest muscles in the body attach to the hip bones, creating pushing-and-pulling forces that can cause some unleveling. A multitude of vector forces placed into this area require our body to have some play built into it to avoid injury. The sacral bone is the keystone of the hip mechanism. We can see in this X-ray how the triangular-shaped bone sits in between the iliac bones.

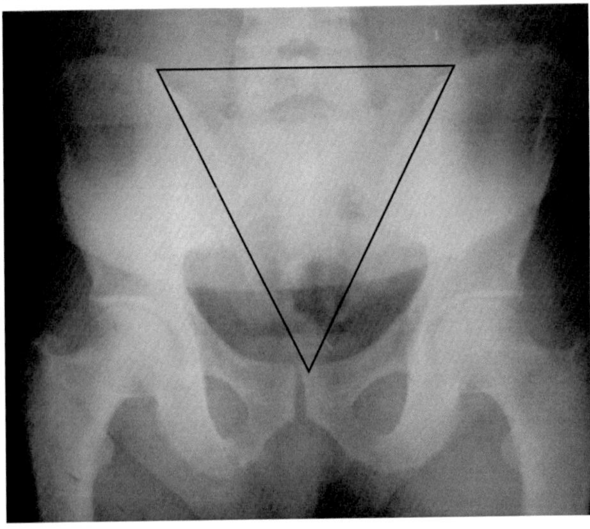

The sacroiliac joint is a common source of problems as we age. This joint is classified as an amphiarthrodial joint. While that is a mouthful, it means the joint is supposed to move a little bit, but not a lot. The joint is supposed to glide slightly with movement of our legs and spine. When this free flowing movement is disrupted, problems start. This is the number one place in the human body that we see fixation. Fixation or subluxation is a condition whereby one boney part gets caught or locked up against another boney part. This fixation can lead to injury, either in the form of strain and swelling of the joint itself, or to any of the muscles or tendons that are associated with the joint in the area. This is where chiropractors shine. SI fixations are reduced almost magically with chiropractic treatments. Hip misalignment and SI joint fixation can be helped with the Big Five treatments. Moving the hip bones to their normal positions reduces stress placed into the connecting structures. Simply inducing a force in the right line of correction breaks the SI joint loose quite nicely.

The hamstrings anchor into the pelvis and limit flexion of the torso. The tighter your hamstrings are, the lesser your pelvic motion. So if you suffer chronic SI joint or pelvic misalignment issues, you might want to concentrate on increasing the flexibility of your hamstrings. Patients that suffer from hypermobility problems of the SI and hip region can benefit by wearing a sacroiliac belt. (**wolfsibelt.com**)

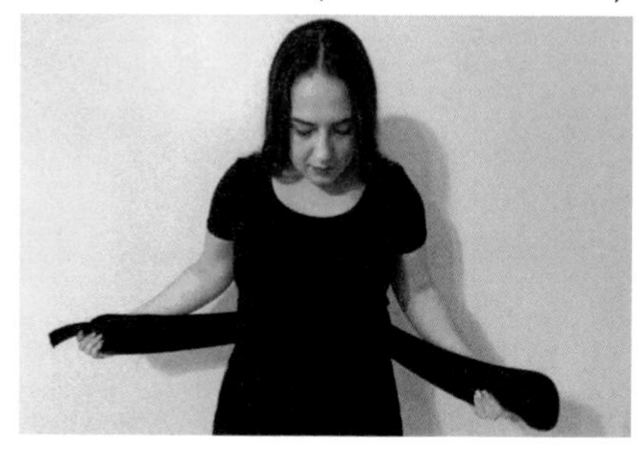

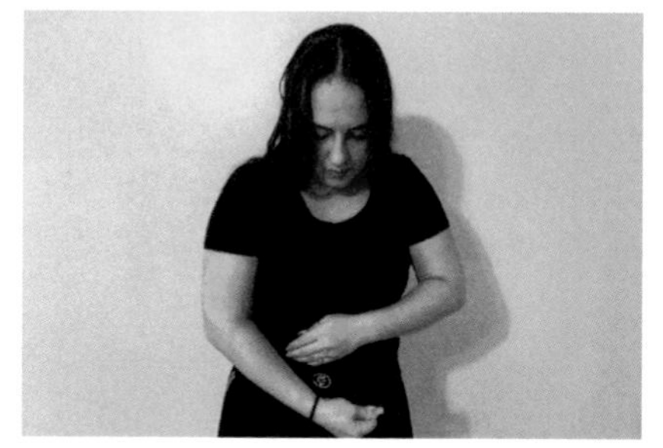

B) Iliotibial Band Syndrome

The iliotibial band (IT band) is a band of tissue that extends from the side of the hip all the way down to the side of the knee. When injured, this thin sheath of tissue will contract or shorten. The tension created can cause discomfort on the side of the knee or over the side of the hip. The anatomy of the body presents a few challenges here. Bursa sacs are the structures that make synovial fluid. Synovial fluid lubricates the joint. The trochanteric bursa is located right over the greater trochanter of the femur bone and right under the IT Band. This particular bone has a bone point called the greater trochanter which can be very sharp or pointed on some people. When the IT Band contracts, it puts downward pressure on the bursa into the point of the greater trochanter, effectively poking or stabbing the bursa. This is called iliotibial band syndrome. Friction is created over the bursa, causing the phenomenon of inflammation known as bursitis.

ILIOTIBIAL BAND SYNDROME

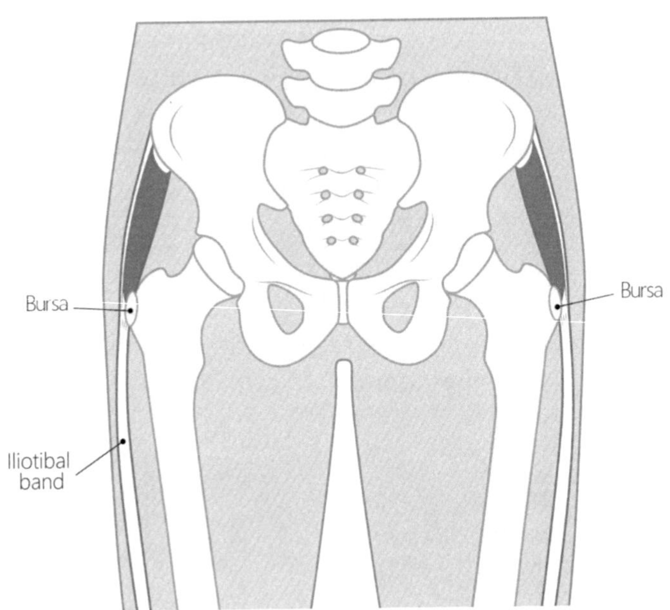

A lot of runners get IT band syndrome from bad biomechanics while running. For example, some runners get into a habit of always running on one side of the road because of traffic patterns. Roads are domed for water runoff. The dome of the road creates an anatomical short leg on the leg that is closest to the inside of the road and a long leg on the one that is on the outside of the road.

Errant biomechanics have to be corrected for recovery from IT band syndrome. Running on a flat surface is important. If someone has an anatomic leg length discrepancy, the same problem could occur. Usually, the leg that is longer will have more traction forces on the IT band, thereby creating more pressure on the bursa. If this is the case, simply putting a heel lift in your shoe on the short leg side can take care of this. (**wolfheellift.com**). Excess pronation of the foot caused by a collapsing arch can cause the same problem. In this case, an orthotic does the trick. (**wolforthotics.com**) Another aggregating factor can be side sleeping. When you have an injured IT band, it's helpful to sleep on your back. The problem with sleeping on the affected side is that the bursa gets squeezed from your body weight. When you sleep with the affected side up, the natural contour of your body shape can put a slight traction load on the IT band. When sleeping on your side, a pillow between your legs can decrease the traction on the IT band, particularly if you are a woman or someone with wider hips. Of course, this means the affected side would sleep in the "up" position while using the pillow between your legs.

To restore the IT band back to its normal length it must be stretched. The pictures below show three different ways you can stretch the IT band. One you can do while laying, another while sitting and yet another while standing. I tell my patients to stretch this band ad nauseum. If you stretch it 1,000 times a day, you will recover quicker then stretching it 100 times a day.

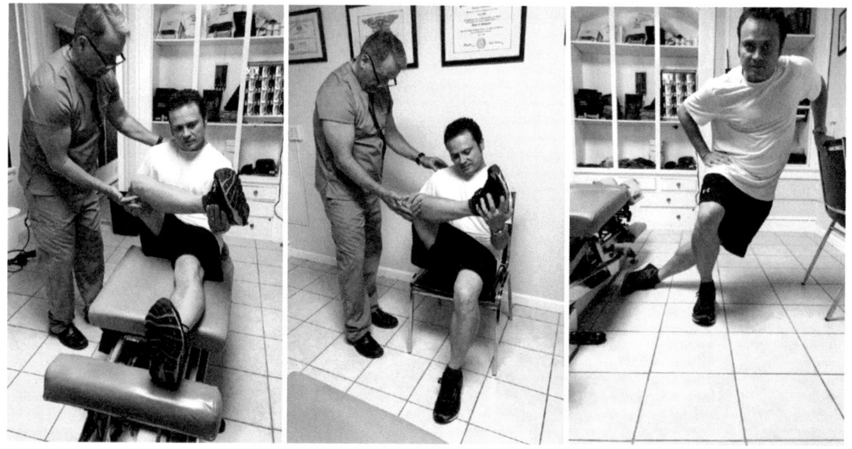

The more you stretch the IT band, the quicker it will recover its length and reduce the stress on the bursa. In a few rare cases, the IT band is restored to its original length, but the bursa is so sore from the friction caused by the tight IT band that you are now left with plain old bursitis. In this case, I refer the patient to an orthopedist to get a steroid injection into the bursa itself. It is very important to have the IT band completely stretched out to its normal length before getting the steroid shot. If the band is still tight, the continual pressure on the bursa will keep it inflamed and the shot won't work.

C) Piriformis Syndrome

The piriformis muscle originates on the hip and inserts into the femur bone. This muscle goes right over the sciatic nerve. The sciatic nerve is the biggest nerve in the body. When there is a contracture of this muscle, the sciatic nerve gets entrapped and the patient will experience pain down his leg.

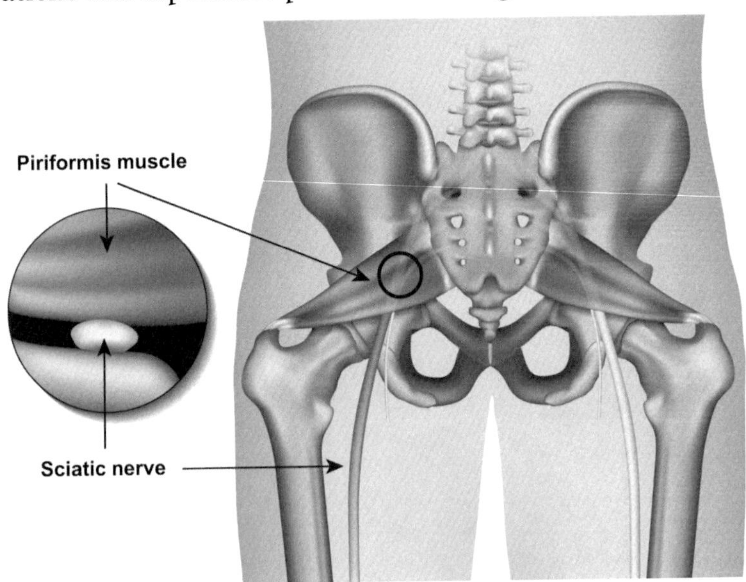

Because the pain radiates down the leg, this condition gets misdiagnosed as a lumbar disc herniation. The causes for contracture of this muscle are numerous. Direct injury to the muscle could cause contracture. Just like with IT band issues, bad training mechanics can be the root of the problem. Leg length discrepancy can trigger piriformis contractures. The first way to treat this problem is to get the piriformis muscle stretched back to its normal length. The following picture shows how to stretch the right piriformis muscle out. It looks very similar to the IT band stretch only the right foot must stay on the ground.

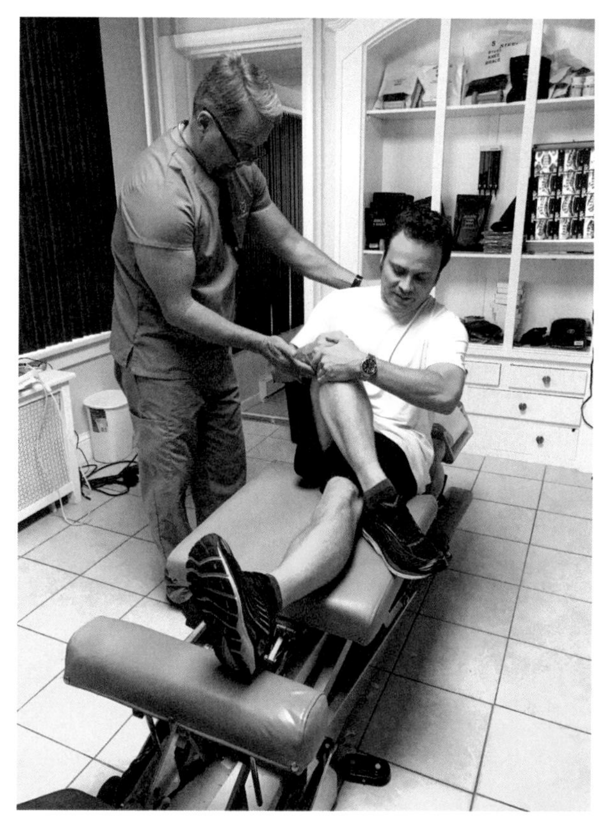

Evaluation of training mechanics would be next. For example, making sure the patient is running on even ground, or checking his shoes to make sure there isn't abnormal wear. Then, evaluate to see if there is a leg length issue. If so, a heel lift does the trick. (**wolfheellift.com**) Furthermore, I always encourage the patient to wear orthotics to help keep stable foot mechanics when walking or running. (**wolforthotics.com**)

Shoulder Disorders

As we age the shoulder presents a lot of challenges with training. To understand the mechanisms of injury, it's helpful to learn the basic anatomy of the shoulder. We will start with bone issues first. We have 3 bones that comprise the shoulder joint; the humerus, scapula, and clavicle.

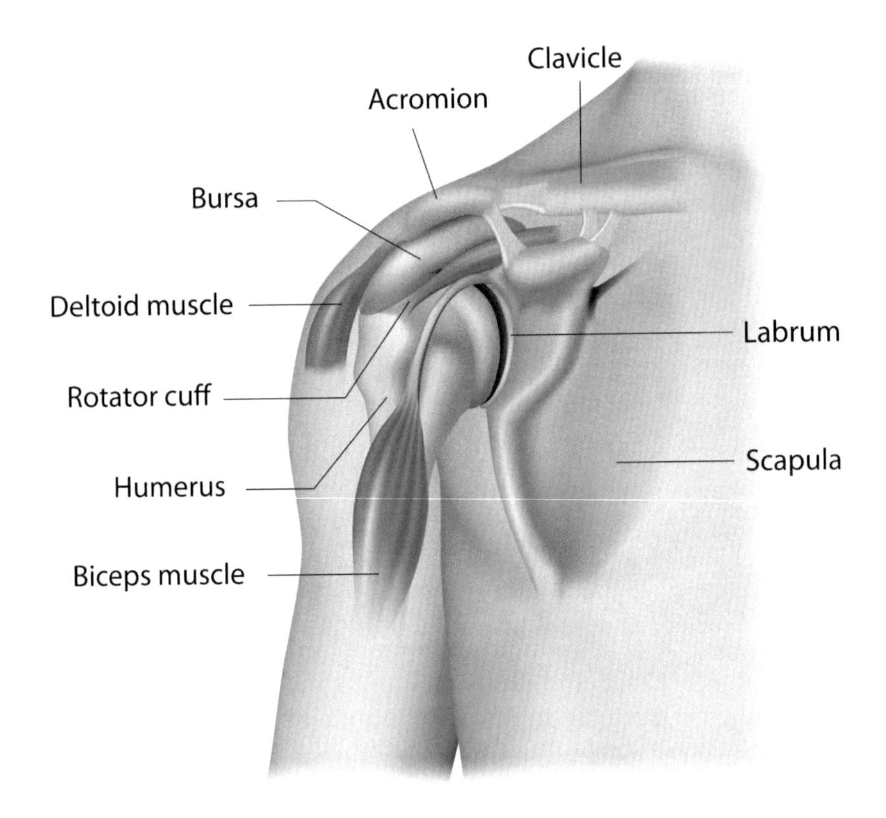

A) Shoulder Dislocation

When the humerus is pulled out of the socket it is called a dislocation. The resulting dislocation is extremely painful and can appear quite gruesome.

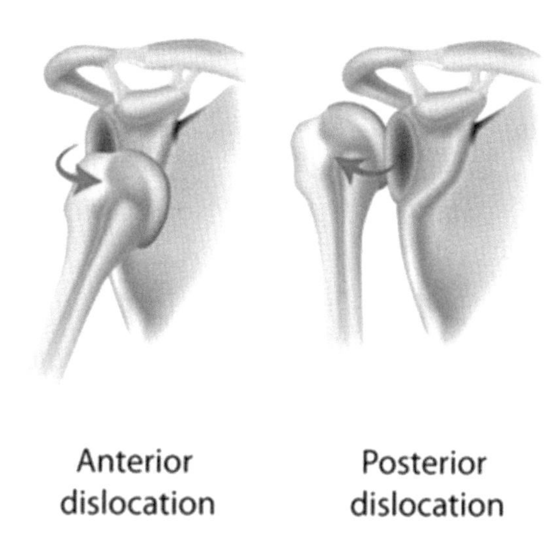

Anterior dislocation

Posterior dislocation

This can be a serious injury. The cause is usually traumatic in nature. Causes that are non-traumatic include dislocations from instability due to extreme laxity of the ligaments or missing ligaments. Usually, people that have a passive dislocation have a history of it happening several times with the most benign incident. There is a technique to reduce the dislocation called the Kocher's maneuver. This reduction of the dislocation can usually be performed safely if the dislocation is from passive activity. This should only be attempted by a health care practitioner with training. The maneuver consists of pulling the arm downward in a superior to inferior fashion. Interestingly, this usually reduces the severe pain the patient is suffering. Next, the arm is externally rotated, abducted, and then the humerus falls right into place.

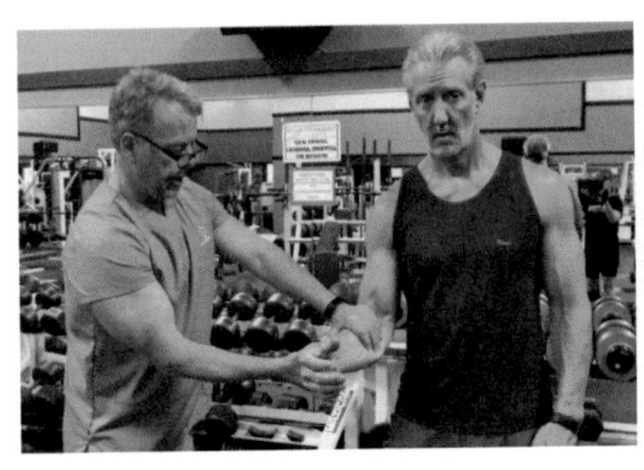

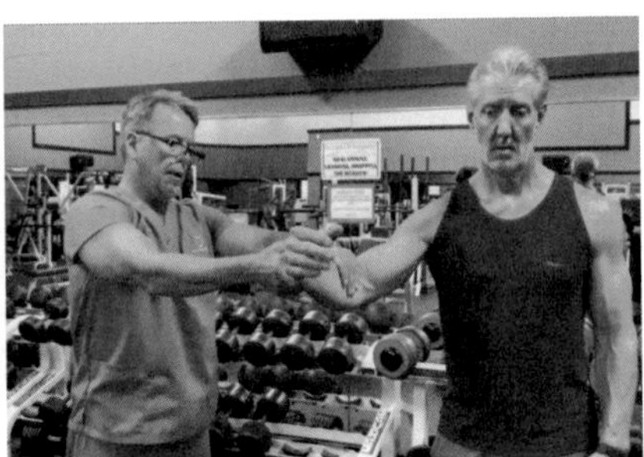

Again, this maneuver should only be attempted by a trained specialist. In cases of traumatic dislocation, this maneuver shouldn't be performed in the field until an X-ray or MRI can rule out complications such as a fracture.

Treatment for shoulder dislocation involves reduction as soon as possible. Immobilization for a very short time in the initial acute phase is advisable, followed by the Big Five treatment for sure. An orthopedist should be consulted to rule out damage that needs surgical repair to avoid potential problems down the road.

B) Shoulder Separation

The collarbone or clavicle forms a joint with the connecting wing bone or scapula. This joint is called the acromioclavicular joint or AC joint. This is a common injury in young athletes involved in contact sports. Traumatic insult to the arm results in a traction force to the joint, causing the acromioclavicular ligament that holds the two bones together to tear. Depending on the severity, the coracoclavicular ligament can tear. Also, separations can occur slowly over time from repetitive microtrauma. For example, a baseball pitcher that has thrown too many innings.

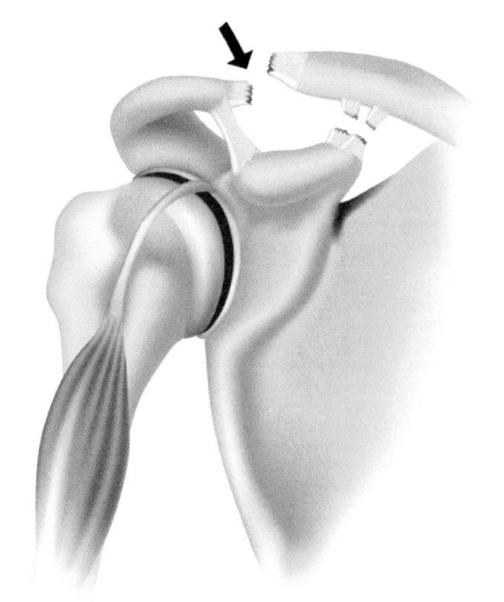

An acute separation produces a lot of pain. In most cases, no surgery needs to be performed. The pain resolves itself in a few weeks. The Big Five treatment is very helpful in managing this one. Unfortunately, there is a cosmetic deformity associated with this injury.

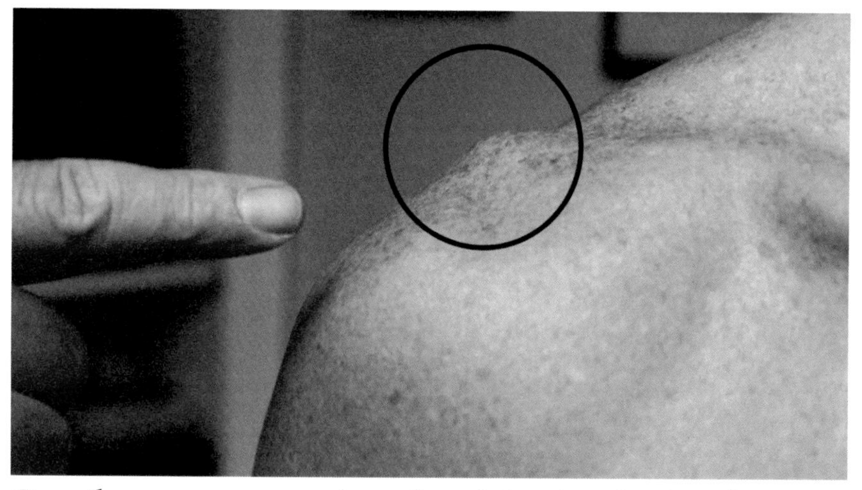

Over the years surgeons have found that just leaving the injury alone results in quicker recovery and decreased incidence of recurrence.

C) Broken Collar Bone

A broken collarbone is usually the direct result of trauma. I see a lot of these injuries with cyclists who take a spill. While the fracture is usually quite painful, treatment is limited to immobilization to reduce pain. The Big Five will speed recovery and can help with the pain. Surprisingly, like with separations, surgeons have found that this injury does better by just leaving it alone. There's more risk with the procedure to reduce it than leaving it be. The downside is that you are left with a cosmetic deformity. As with any fracture, check with your chiropractor or orthopedist to have it properly evaluated. Typically, it's a self-limiting problem. I had a patient that fractured his collarbone while training for a triathlon. He was disappointed because he had to compete next week. To my surprise, he asked if he could still compete. I told him he wasn't going to make the fracture worse and advised him that it would be shear torture to do the swimming part of the event. He did and it was. He is one tough mother!

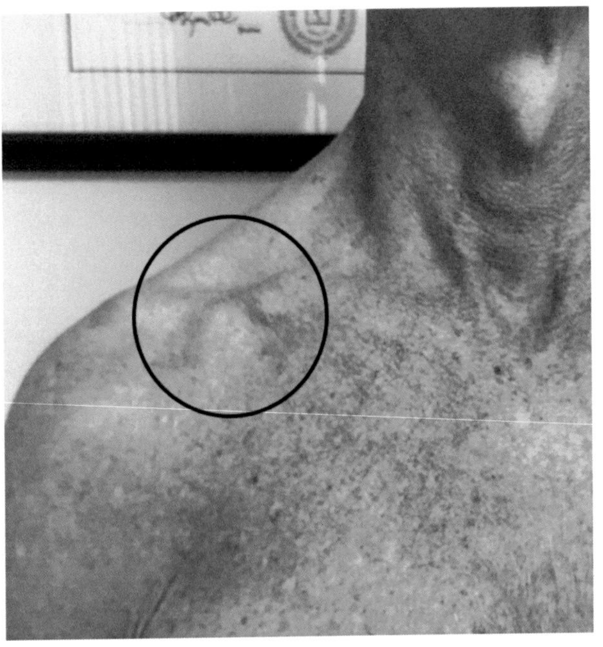

D) Labral Tear

The labrum is the female part of the shoulder joint that joins the arm in the socket. This strong fibrocartilage helps with stabilization of the humeral head in the shoulder joint. Injury to the labrum can be caused by dislocation, microtrauma from translation deformity, and repetitive throwing activity. Another common way of injuring the labrum is a slip or fall. The natural instinct is to break your fall with your arm. The resulting telescopic force into the shoulder joint can tear the labrum.

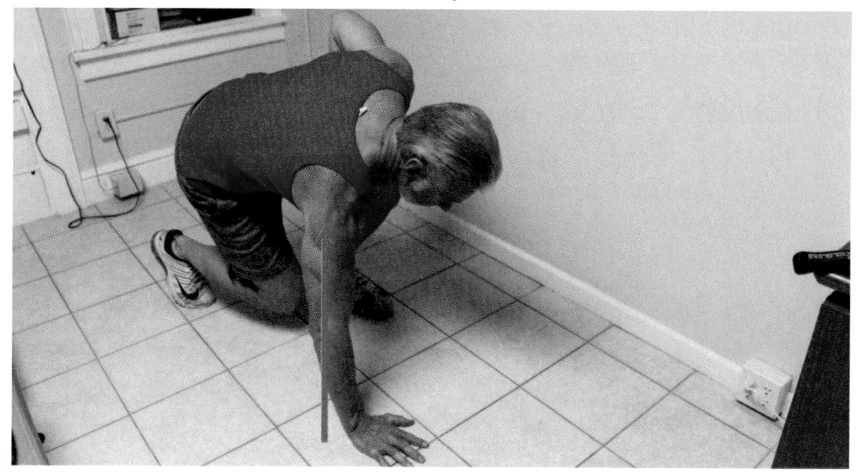

Symptoms include anything from mild to severe pain. Mild pain is usually an indication of strain and not necessarily a tear. If there is severe pain with simple movements of the shoulder there could be a tear. Depending on the severity, this one can heal on its own. It's important with damage to the labrum to evaluate the cause. If it's from translation deformity problems, it's paramount to strengthen the surrounding rotator cuff muscles. By doing this, you use the muscles to help stabilize the loose joint. In the next section, we're going to discuss rotator cuff injuries and how to rehabilitate these muscles. Using the Big Five approach helps by bringing blood to the tissues, which aides in recovery. Sometimes steroid injections can do wonders with this injury. If a severe injury occurs and the pain does not resolve, shoulder surgery is usually required.

E) Rotator Cuff Injuries

This is by far the most common source of shoulder pain in the 40-plus crowd. The pain could be anything from a nagging toothache-type pain to severe, sharp debilitating pain. The rotator cuff is comprised of four muscles that encapsulate the humeral head. They are known as the SITS muscles: the supraspinatus, infraspinatus, teres minor, and subscapularis.

Rotator Cuff Muscles

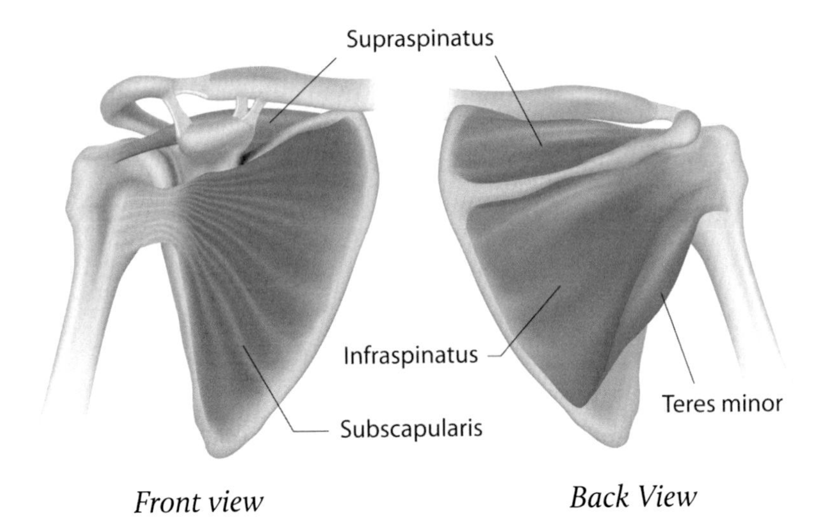

Front view *Back View*

These muscles are responsible for rotational movements of your arm and abduction motions. Before we go any further, I want to be clear as to what abduction is because we are going to use the term a lot in this section. It's the motion we make when we lift our arm to the side. The picture below shows our model abducting his arm.

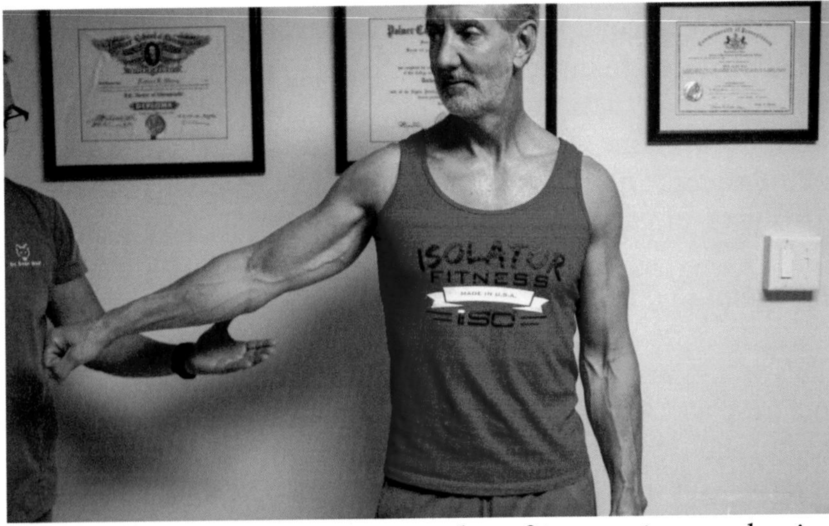

The shoulder anatomy presents a lot of interesting mechanical situations with the arm. The hook shaped acromion process can jab into the bicipital tendon and the supraspinatus tendon with simple abduction moves.

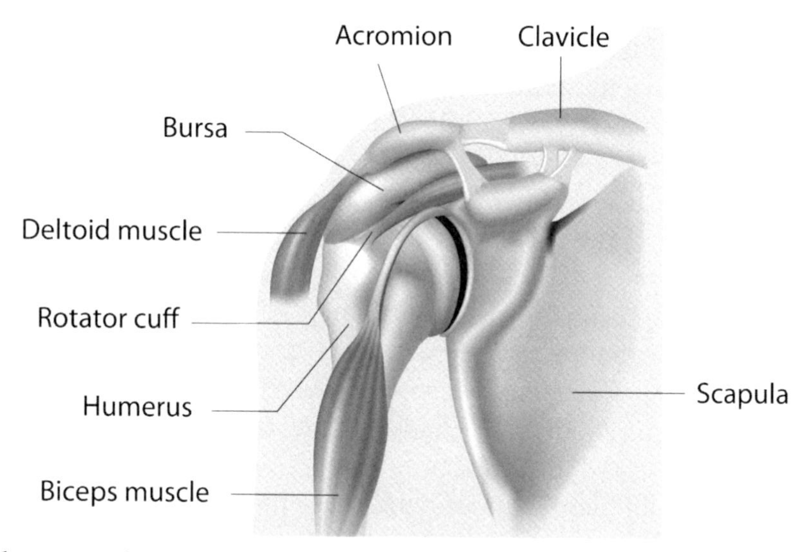

The space between the acromion and the humerus is called the acromial humeral (AH) interval. The spacing here is the key to injury. The following X-ray on the left shows a normal AH interval.

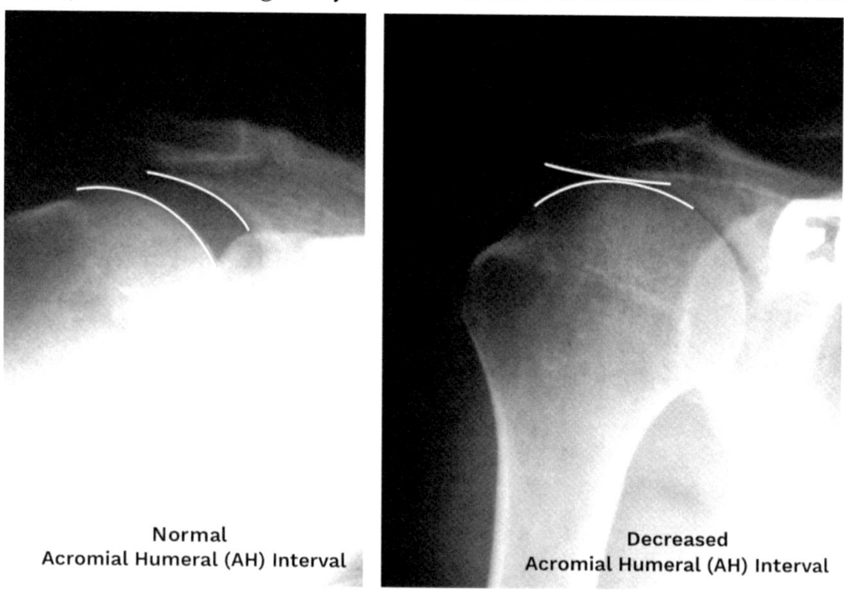

The X-ray on the right shows a decrease in the AH interval. When this space decreases, the bursa gets smashed, the bicipital and supraspinatus tendons get pinched, and impingement occurs. Now imagine what would happen when you lift your arm (abduct) to the side? All those tissues would get pinched even more. You might ask, "What causes a decrease in space?" It can be a congenital anomaly caused by a large or hook shaped acromion process. Most of the time, it is a slow decrease in space caused by progressive decreased rotator cuff muscle strength. Interestingly, the weaker the cuff, the further decrease in space. The less space, the more pressure on the cuff muscles. The more pressure on the cuff muscles, the weaker the cuff becomes. This is a snowball running down a mountain. It just keeps getting worse, and it all started with weakness. How does weakness occur? As we get older, we naturally develop a systemic decrease in muscle mass throughout our entire body. During normal activity, we still use our chest and arm muscles. When you see how we exercise the rotator cuff, you'll understand these motions aren't common with normal activities. Thus, it's imperative to intentionally focus on this area for strengthening.

With every muscle group, we have balance. An agonist and antagonist, a ying and yang. For example, when we are sitting or standing, there are muscles that pull us forward and muscles that pull us backward. There are muscles that pull us to the right and muscles that pull us to the left. If one set of muscles is weaker than its counterpart, the stronger muscles pull the anatomy to the strong side. Now imbalance has occurred. Anytime there is imbalance, there is a predisposition to injury. Since the rotator cuff muscles basically pull the shoulder back and down, the antagonist muscles pull the shoulder up and front. Just a simple visual inspection can diagnose rotator cuff injury. The following picture shows a rotator cuff injury. You can clearly see the patient's right shoulder is forward and elevated as compared to the left.

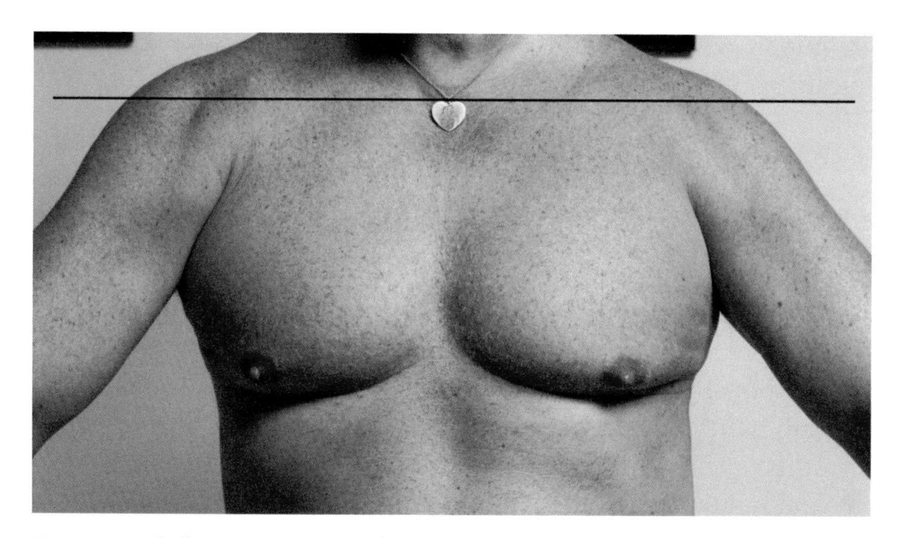

Strains of the rotator cuff are simple to rehabilitate. Injury to the rotator cuff tendons are a little trickier. If there is a simple strain, exercises can completely fix the problem in 4-6 weeks. When exercised, these tissues respond quickly. Tendon injuries can take longer and often result in tendinopathies like we spoke of in Chapter 7. We will go over each rotator cuff muscle and how to specifically strengthen each individually. Remember from Chapter 7, a tendonosis diagnosis means that sufferers need to perform eccentric cuff contractions which then apply resisted negative force into the muscle's normal range of motion. I know this can be confusing or hard to visualize. Don't worry, I made videos showing how to do all of these exercises in both concentric and eccentric lines of correction at **DrDeanWolf.com**. Following exercise, the Big Five treatment is still the best way to enhance recovery and reduce pain. One of the hallmark symptoms of rotator cuff injuries is night pain. The reason is that disuse gives the body the chance to swell. Often, patients relate laying in bed and their shoulder feels a toothache-like pain. During the day, we move and we walk and this physical motion creates some dispersal of edema or swelling. It's almost like squeezing water out of a rag. Sometimes doing rotator cuff exercises can be like taking an aspirin. Just working the tendons and muscles takes the discomfort away. It's very important not to put your shoulder in a sling when there is a rotator cuff injury – it can lead to a frozen shoulder, which we will explain in the next section. First, let's discuss each rotator cuff muscle individually.

1. Supraspinatus

This is the top rotator cuff muscle and the one that's most commonly injured. Because of its location, it's usually the one that gets creamed by the acromion process during abduction movement. Also, it's more prone to compromise due to the fact it's responsible for initiating abduction of the arm. If you're having pain or discomfort lifting your arm to the side, chances are this is the guy that's beat up. Exercising this muscle looks a little unusual. The key is to internally rotate your arms as far as you can. Then lift your arm at a 45° angle, halfway between the front of you and the side of you. Then only lift your arm 45° away from your body. When I do this exercise with two dumbbells, I think of myself coming away from my body like a letter "V." It's a short, very specific motion. Be careful to do this exactly right. Do not lift your arms higher than 45 degrees.

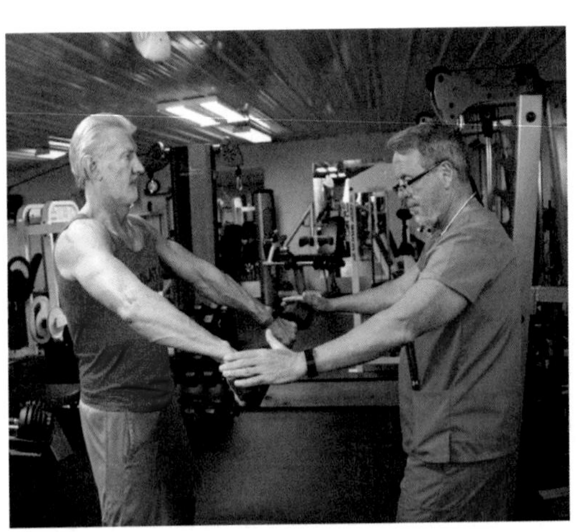

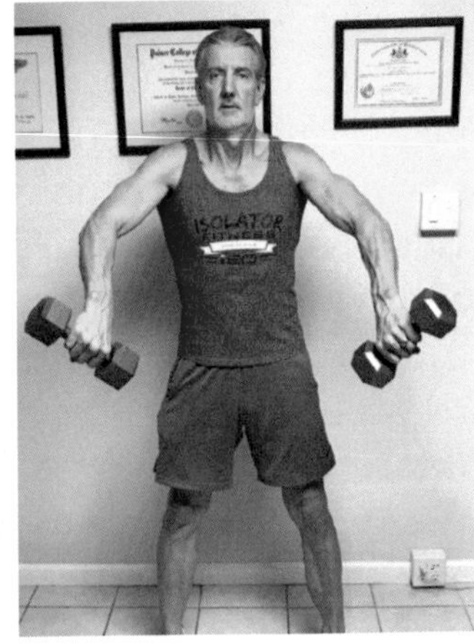

Remember, we don't want to strengthen the antagonist muscles. I love using exercise bands for this exercise. I feel a constant force, and I can wrap them up and put them in my pocket to take them anywhere (**wolfbands.com**).

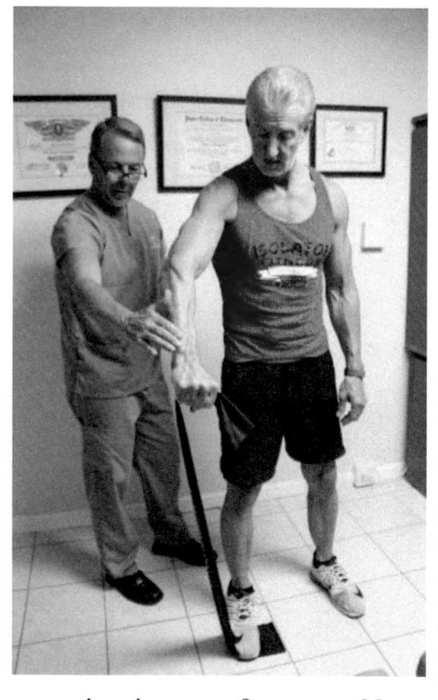

2. Infraspinatus and Teres Minor

I grouped these two muscles together because they work synergistically to externally rotate the arm. When I exercise these muscles, the motion is the reverse of arm wrestling. When doing this motion, it's important to keep your elbow at your side. They call it the rotator cuff because these muscles rotate your arm. This is achieved by keeping the elbow fixed at your side. The other thing you have to watch out for with this one is not to go through a long range of motion. You want to exercise in a 90° range. You start this exercise with your hand against your stomach. Then externally rotate until your fist is pointing straight ahead. Don't continue to externally rotate any further. This is another great exercise to do with exercise bands. (**wolfbands.com**)

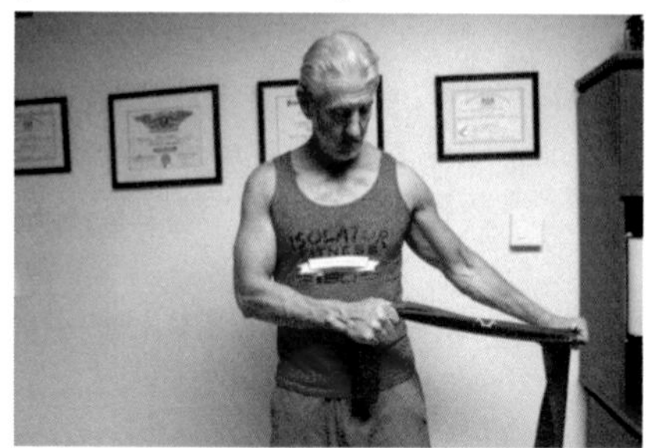

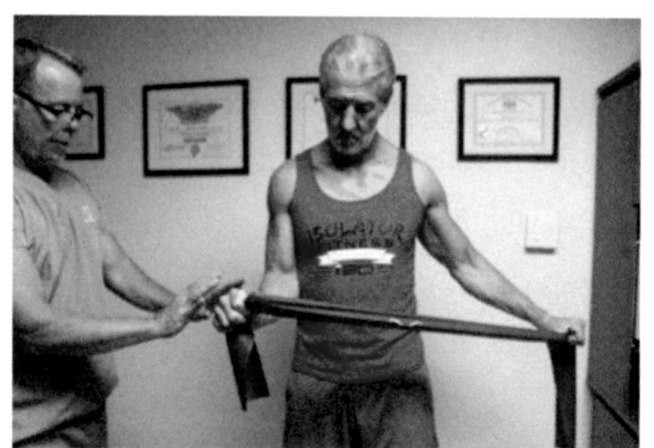

The band's progressive resistance helps get the maximum work out of this muscle and tendon. Check out the videos for these exercises at **DrDeanWolf.com**.

3. Subscapularis

This is the least injured cuff muscle by far. In fact, I've only seen this one tear with high velocity trauma. The subscapularis is usually not a victim of microtrauma. This muscle performs an internal rotation of your arm – the motion that you would use during an arm wrestling match. If you have discomfort or pain in your shoulder during internal rotation, you probably have injury to the labrum and not the subscapularis. If pain occurs, discontinue the exercise and call your chiropractor or orthopedist. To exercise the subscapularis, you would do just the opposite motion of the infraspinatus and teres minor movements.

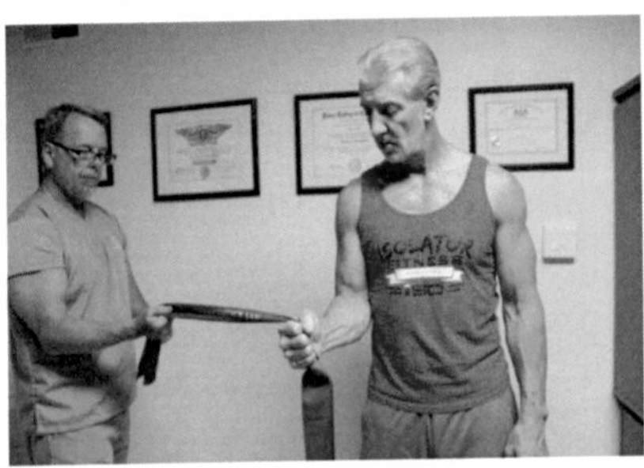

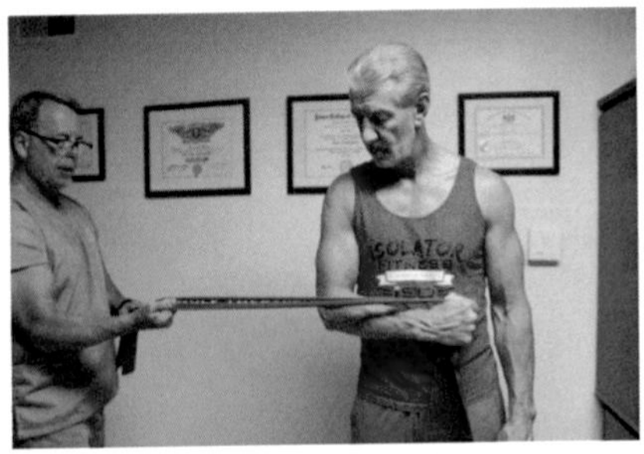

If you have no rotator cuff problems after age fifty, chances are you have an extraordinary shoulder capsule. It's so common to injure these structures one way or another after age 50, especially if you still play some sports or work out at the gym. I tell my patients to find time for a shoulder day once a week in the gym. If you follow this advice, your performance in a variety of activities will be enhanced. You'll hit a golf ball further and throw a bowling ball harder. Your serve in tennis will be hotter. It could take 80 newtons of force to throw a baseball. It takes a lot more force to stop the arm that is throwing that baseball. Your body will never let you throw an object harder than it can stop the arm at the end of a throwing motion. If it did, your arm would dislocate. The stronger your decelerators are, the more your body will allow you to accelerate. Want to hit a golf ball 10 yards farther? Strengthen your rotator cuff muscles.

F) Frozen Shoulder

Frozen shoulder is also known as adhesive capsulitis of the shoulder. Simply put, the body turns the shoulder into stone. We could go into the complexities of glycosylation and the mechanisms of how collagen fibers can form at unprecedented speed that causes the shoulder to freeze. Instead, let's focus on the factors that can predispose you to this condition.

For years, rotator cuff injuries were misdiagnosed as strains and sprains. The doctor often treated these by simply putting your arm in a sling. Separated shoulders and dislocated shoulders alike were treated similarly. Rotator cuff surgery and traumatic situations can put you in a situation whereby the shoulder must be immobilized. Because of disuse and the immobilization of the shoulder caused by the sling, the structures lack the blood supply needed to heal the tissue, thereby facilitating the formation of a frozen shoulder. Other factors that increase the probability of this happening are diabetes, thyroid dysfunction, and autoimmune disorders.

The most important thing to keep in mind with any shoulder injury is to not immobilize it for any extended period of time. With the exception of surgical situations, don't use a sling. You need to move your shoulder as soon as you are able. The quicker you use it, the less likely you are to lose it. Of course, shoulder surgery will limit your ability to use your arm. Follow your surgeon's advice on when to start to use the arm. The quicker the better. Ice and other treatments in the Big Five are very helpful in any shoulder injury and particularly with frozen shoulder.

G) Bursitis and Impingement Syndrome

I lumped these two disorders together because they are closely tied. We discussed impingement problems with the supraspinatus rotator cuff muscle. Impingement syndrome (swimmer's shoulder) in the context of rotator cuff weakness means that there is muscle entrapment. Bursitis is usually a manifestation of the impingement. The bursa sits right under the acromion process of the scapula. When this area gets pinched, the bursa gets smashed and consequently inflamed.

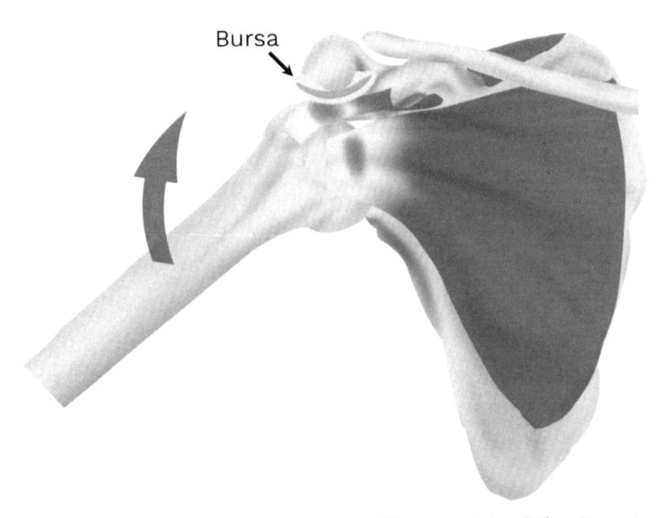

Simply strengthening the rotator cuff gets rid of the impingement and consequential bursitis. This usually works quite nicely, although I've had a few stubborn cases where the bursa wanted to stay inflamed. In those instances, I refer my patients to an orthopedist for a steroid injection. The injection gets them over the hump quickly; however, the underlying impingement must be resolved. Strengthening the rotator cuff muscles, especially the supraspinatus, opens the space in the exact place where the pinch occurs. Just like with piriformis syndrome and trochanteric bursitis, the bursa stays inflamed if the causation is not removed. The Big Five treatment helps reduce recovery time and pain. A TENS unit can help reduce the night pain associated with this condition (**wolftensunit.com**).

Biceps and Triceps Injuries

A) Biceps and Triceps Tendinitis and Tendonosis

Your biceps and your triceps are your proverbial guns. Even guns break once in a while. Tendinitis can occur and is easily treated with the Big Five. The biggest threat to the bicep and tricep is tendonosis. As discussed in Chapter 7, tendinopathies can be treated and resolved quite easily with eccentric contractions. If you suffer from this, refer back to Chapter 7 for the basic principle. Personally, I have suffered from tendonosis of the long head of my right bicep. Just to refresh you on how stubborn these injuries are, allow me to engage you in a self-deprecating story. I had noticed some bicep discomfort after doing a heavy hammer curl routine. When bowling in a league later that week, I experienced significant pain in the front of my arm when I threw the ball. Since it was the last night of my bowling league, I didn't think much of it. No big deal – bowling season was over and golf season was beginning. I didn't have a problem with the bicep while playing golf. 5 months later, bowling season started again. My first shot of the night, I felt a sharp pain in the distal part of my bicep at my elbow that sent me to the moon. The last shot of the night hurt just as badly as the first. It was a long night! I told my buddies to get me a sub for the next month because I knew I had some work to do. Every other day for 4 weeks, I drilled my right bicep with eccentric contractions. In 1 month, my bicep was like brand new.

These tendonosis issues will not resolve themselves. When faced with this injury, most people just quit the activity. All they have to do is force the body to rebuild the tissue and they will be back in action again! (you can find videos for bicep and tricep tendonosis on **DrDeanWolf.com**)

B) Bicep and Tricep Avulsions

This is another common injury for those over 50 – or even 40. An avulsion is when part of the muscle and tendon tear right out of the bone. Usually when suffering from this injury, you will hear an audible pop that's pretty distinctive followed by severe pain and loss of strength. This condition needs to be evaluated by an orthopedist. In most cases the condition is self-limiting, meaning the pain and dysfunction will resolve on its own. That doesn't mean the tendon will glue itself back into the bone. What it means is that you might have only lost 10% of your muscle.

After the pain subsides most find there is little loss of function. You will usually be left with a cosmetic change that looks like a lump. With bicipital avulsions, it sometimes looks like you have a Popeye muscle.

With most of these cases, the cause is directly related to tendonosis. When the tendon degrades and becomes brittle, it is more likely to crack and tear away from the bone. Most people with avulsion injuries had warning signs that were not addressed.

Elbow

For the most part, the elbow is a very stable joint. There are limited problems with ligament and translation deformities here, although they can occur. Sometimes bursitis finds its way into the olecranon anatomy, where the elbow is located. The most common injuries to this area are epicondylitis and fractures.

A) Fractures

Fractures usually occur to the radial head, where the radius meets the elbow. Typically they occur during falls. As with most fractures, they must be evaluated by an orthopedic surgeon to see if intervention is needed. However, most times the injury will need immobilization and time. Usually, with radial head fractures, the patient will lose about fifteen degrees of extension of their arm. Functionally, this is inconsequential.

B) Tendinitis and Tendonosis

Epicondylitis is tendinitis of the elbow and is a frequent reason to visit the doctor's office. We used epicondylitis as our poster child for Chapter 7, dealing with tendinitis and tendonosis. If you have this common elbow problem, refer back to Chapter 7 for more detail in resolving this condition. Most cases of tennis elbow and bowlers elbow after 40 are a function of a tendinopathy and are truly tendonosis. Bracing with a counter brace (**wolfelbowbrace.com**) is extremely helpful in managing pain.

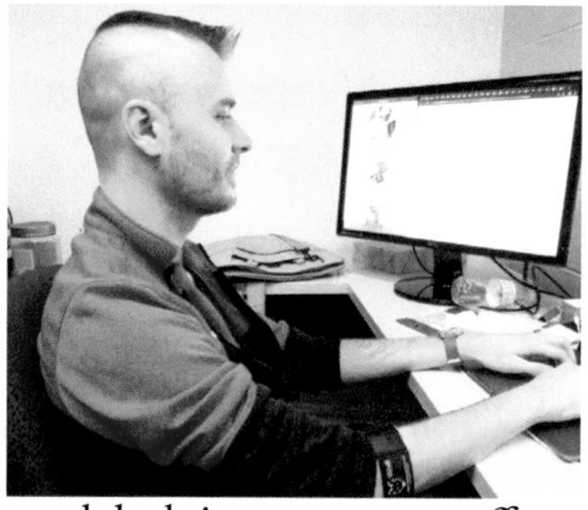

If you are unable to maintain your workout routine because of pain in the elbow when gripping a weight, try the Isolator from *Isolator Fitness* (**isolatorfitness.com**). This tool will keep you working out without pain until resolution of the injury. The following pictures show our model doing rotator cuff exercises with the Isolator. When suffering epicondylitis, these exercises would be practically impossible because of the pain experienced while gripping.

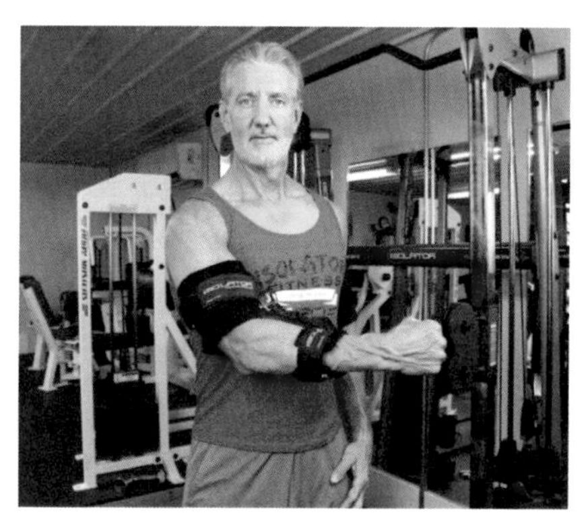

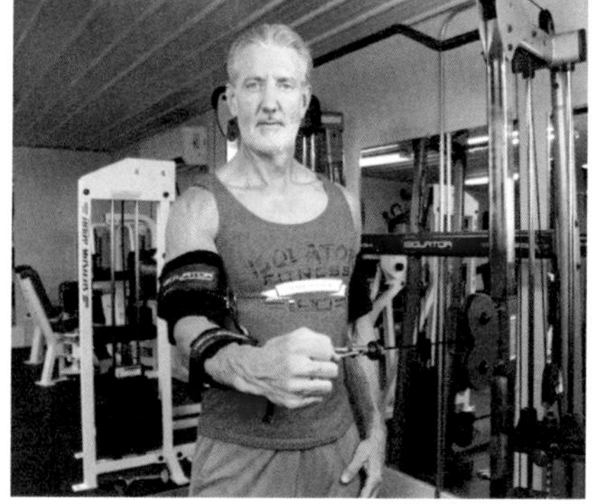

C) Ulnar Nerve Entrapment (Impingement)

On the middle side of the elbow, there is a channel called the ulnar notch. This is where the ulnar nerve passes. There is a ligament that traverses this groove. If this ligament gets tight or the channel itself is congenitally shallow, pressure on the nerve can occur. Ulnar nerve entrapment can occur in the shoulder or in the pinky side of the wrist. When this happens, you will find yourself with numbness or tingling into your pinky and ring finger.

Ulnar Nerve Impingement

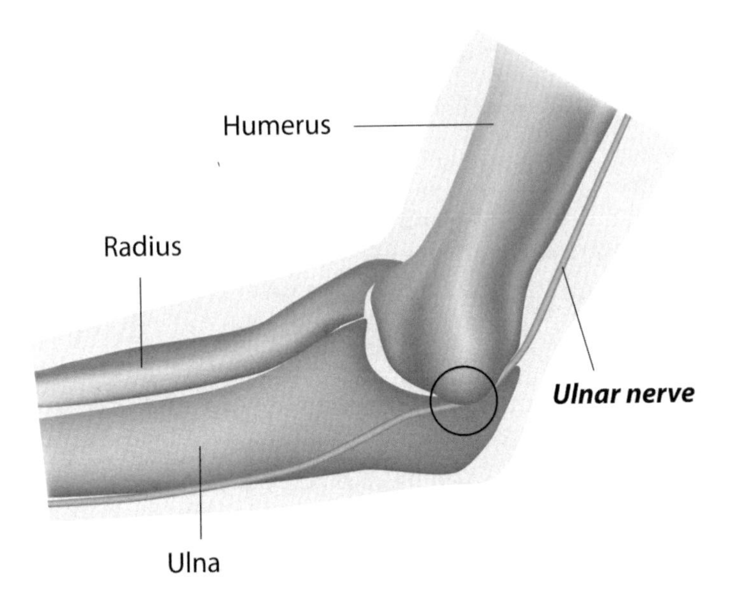

Still the most common site of entrapment is the cubital tunnel. This is the home of the so called "funny bone." Most of us have hit that spot on occasion. When there's pressure in that area, it can be problematic for people that drive for a living or sit in a chair with their elbow on an armrest. When there's already underlying narrowing of the cubital tunnel, the simple pressure exerted by the weight of your arm on an armrest can create a lot of pins and needles. Like all entrapment conditions, the Big Five treatments are not usually effective. Unfortunately, to relieve the pressure, surgery is the best option for this condition.

Wrist

A) Wrist Strains

The wrist is comprised of eight small carpal bones. Motion in the wrist is diverse with circumferential, flexion, extension, and lateral movements. Because there's a bunch of tiny bones with ligaments and cartilage between them, there's a lot of places injuries can hide. Fractures aside, ligament injuries find their way into the wrist area because of its varying range of motion and frequent movement. Treatment of these injuries depends on severity and loss of function. If the pain is mild and loss of function is limited, wrapping the wrist is a great way of making up for the loss of stability from ligament damage (**wolfwristwrap.com**) A wrist wrap can give you added stability, enabling you to still work out and play sports. Personally, I love wearing wrist wraps when I work out. The wrist is much stronger structurally in flexion versus extension. When wrapping the wrist, it should be in a neutral position or slightly flexed for maximum protection.

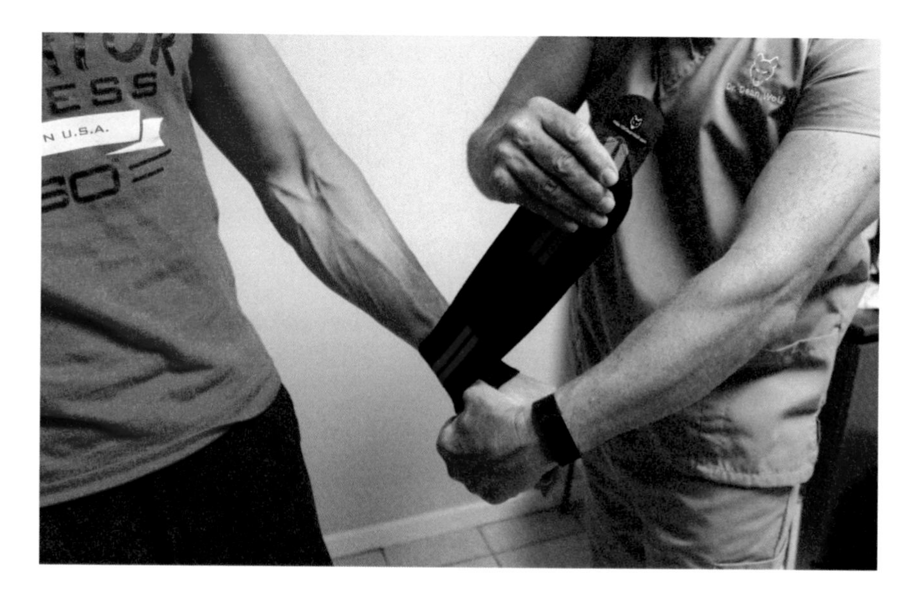

Of the wrist injuries I've seen, the mechanics behind techniques are among the most common sources of problems. For example, to avoid injury when doing a simple rotator cuff exercise, make sure the wrists are static without any movement. Some people with rotator cuff injuries want to extend their wrist as they externally rotate. This puts an inordinate load on the ligaments and cartilage which predisposes them to consequential injuries. The following picture shows the patient using bad technique. The wrist should never extend like shown in the following picture.

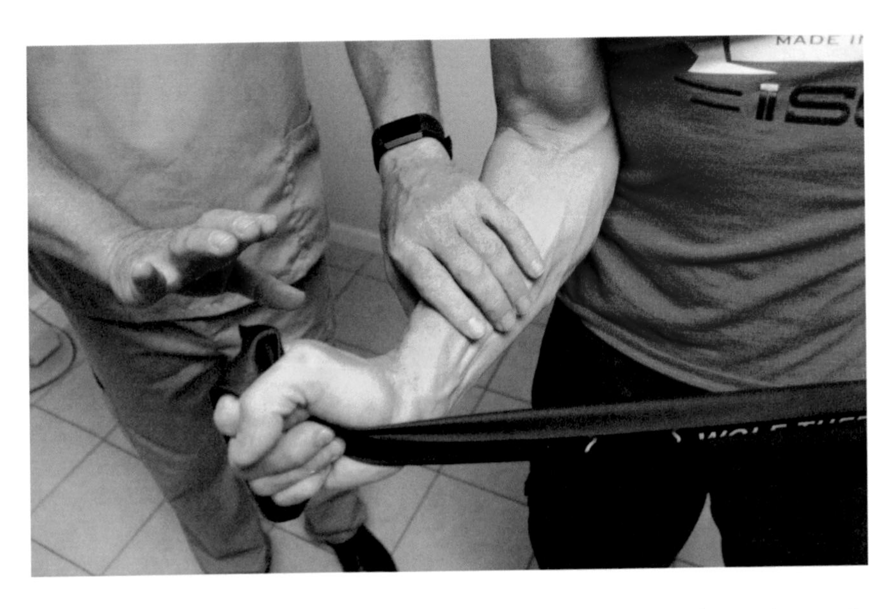

Another cause of injury to the wrist is pure physics. The wrist can't support the heavy weight of some exercises. For example, when doing dumbbell shrugs, we can easily handle heavy weights to work the traps. But the wrists are the weak link in the kinetic chain. I recommend using *ISOGRIPPS*™(**isogripps.com**) when using heavy dumbbells routines to avoid wrist injury. This is my single favorite workout aid and my gym bag is never without it. I've been using this great tool for 5 years. My fiancé is always stealing them from me. We both love to use them when we work out.

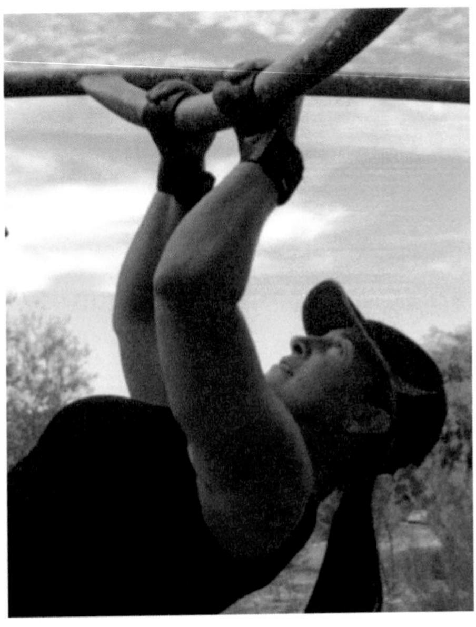

B) Carpal Tunnel Syndrome

Carpal tunnel syndrome (CTS) is the most prevalent of the wrist conditions. The wrist is made up of several bones that have a fibrous bridge called the flexor retinaculum. This bridge forms a tunnel underneath called the carpal tunnel. This is where the median nerve passes. The median nerve is most associated with CTS and its nerve innervation covers the thumb, index finger, middle finger, and the thumb-side half of the ring finger.

If there's pressure on this nerve, you will experience numbness or tingling in the fingers. Women are affected by this disorder more than men, most likely due to having a smaller carpal tunnel. This condition is a combination of how you are built coupled by microtrauma. Most people with this condition have repetitive use jobs that entail a lot of motion in the wrist. Over time, thickening of the structures can cause more pressure on the tunnel. Swelling from overuse can also be a factor. The onset is usually gradual. Symptoms usually start at night when in bed. Patients complain that they wake up with cold, numb, and tingly hands. When shaking their hands out, the feeling comes back. The reason this occurs while sleeping is that we tend to sleep with our hands in a flexed position.

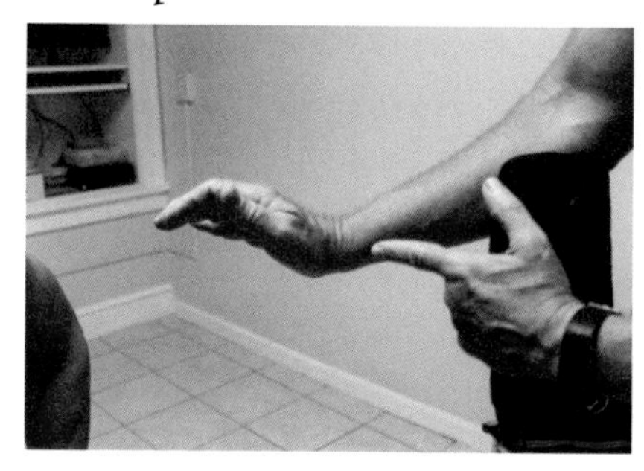

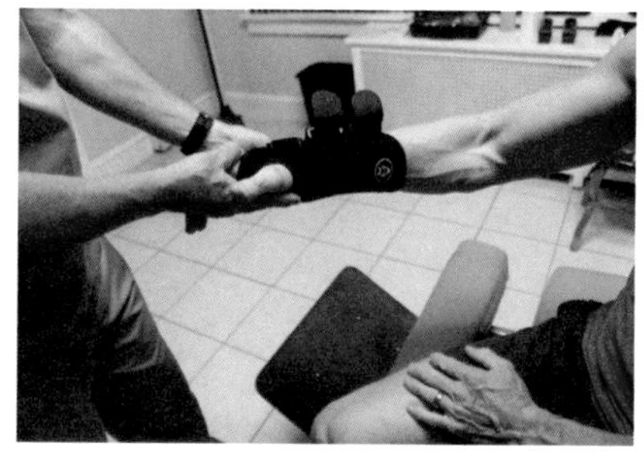

Treatment using the Big Five is not useful for nerve entrapment problems. Decompressing the nerve with a brace can really help. A CTS extension brace can be worn at night to prevent flexion of the wrist from occurring when sleeping. What the brace does is keep the wrist in a neutral or slightly extended position. This allows more room for the median nerve to get through the tunnel.

In a lot of cases, a simple investment in this brace eliminates the problem. (**wolfcarpalbrace.com**)

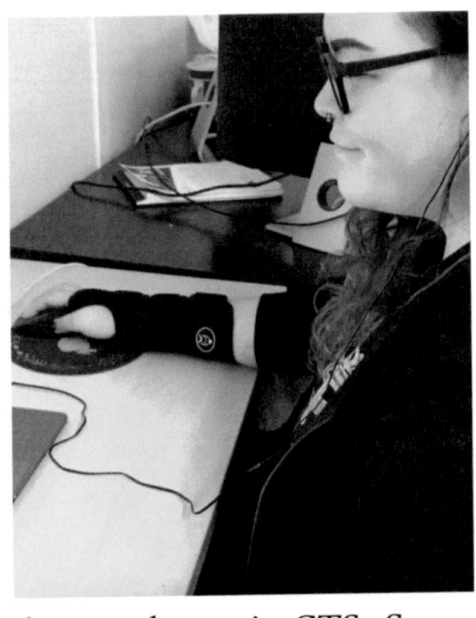

If you have a job that entails a lot of repetitive motions or puts your wrists in flexion for long periods of time, like driving or at a keyboard all day, simply wearing the brace can give you symptomatic relief enabling you to be able to work.

Another thing the CTS brace does is differentiate three things – one being that if the brace gives you relief, it's safe to say the numbness is CTS. Secondly, if the brace doesn't give you relief, you could have a pinched nerve in your elbow, shoulder, or neck. Lastly, if there's no relief, it can mean you have a nasty case of CTS that will probably need decompression surgery. If surgery is needed, the outcome is usually successful. Weakness is something to look for. Remember, loss of function, not pain, is the gold standard of neurosurgery. The primary signs of this loss of function are a loss of muscle mass and strength. If it gets to this point, you probably need surgery. If you suspect you have CTS and you've noticed shrinkage of the muscles of your thumb and palm area, you must get evaluated right away. If atrophy of the muscle occurs, the damage could be permanent.

A clinical examination includes the Tinel tap test, where the doctor taps on the median nerve over the carpal tunnel. If tingling is reproduced, you know you have a winner.

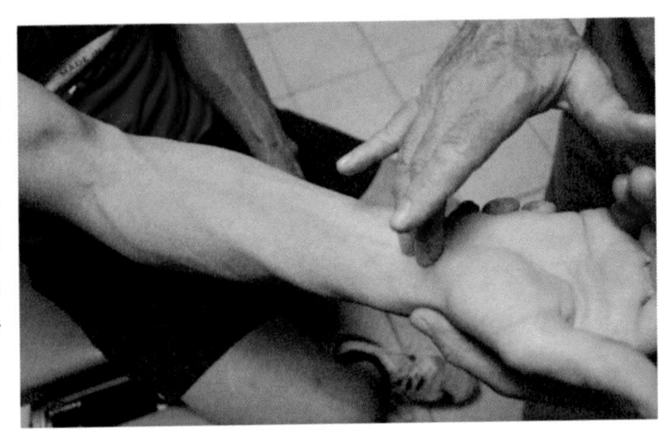

Another test is called Phalen's maneuver. The doctor puts your hands against each other in extreme flexion. This closes the carpal tunnel. If tingling occurs, you likely have CTS.

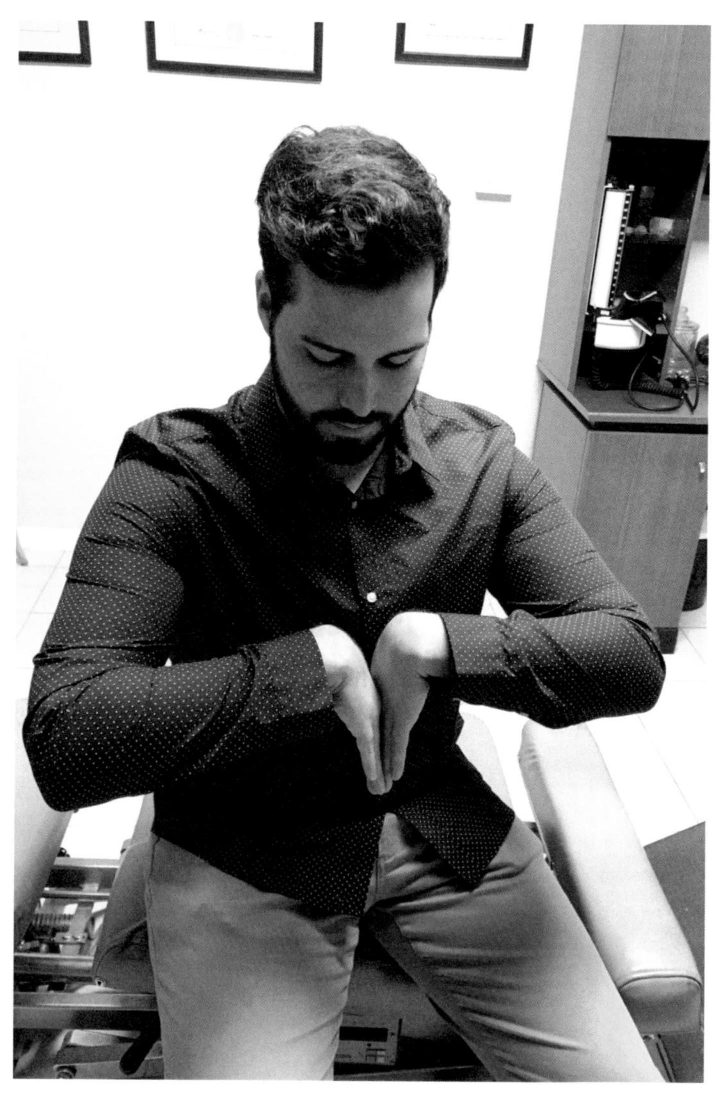

If these tests are positive, you should be referred to an electrodiagnostic specialist. He will perform a nerve conduction velocity test. A nerve conduction velocity test (NCV) will unequivocally diagnose whether or not you have CTS.

Finger Disorders

A) Osteoarthritis

The most common problem with our fingers as we age is osteoarthritis due to wear and tear. The symptoms include stiffness and pain and noticeable bends and bumps at the joints.

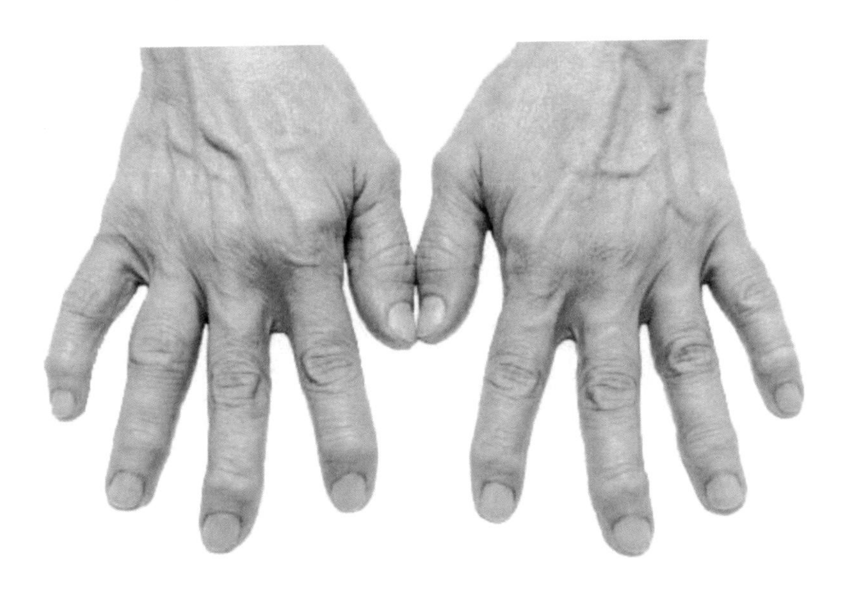

Trauma and repetitive-use causations are common. General aging of the joint's soft tissue components results in the degeneration of the cartilage. Icing and NSAIDs are very helpful in managing the symptoms. Using a natural anti-inflammatory can be helpful. I like turmeric with ginger for these patients. (**wolftumeric.com**) I also really like this glucosamine formula and it makes sense to take it everyday. (**wolfjointrebuild.com**)

B) Rheumatoid Arthritis

This condition is more complicated than generic osteoarthritis. This is an autoimmune problem, meaning the body recognizes its own tissue as being an invader. The body's systems attack the tissue in an effort to get rid of it. This is an inflammation-based disorder; therefore, stopping the inflammation helps manage the symptoms. Ice and NSAIDs can help, but treatment using prescription steroids works the best during the acute phases of this disorder. Diagnosis is accomplished through characteristic X-ray findings and blood work.

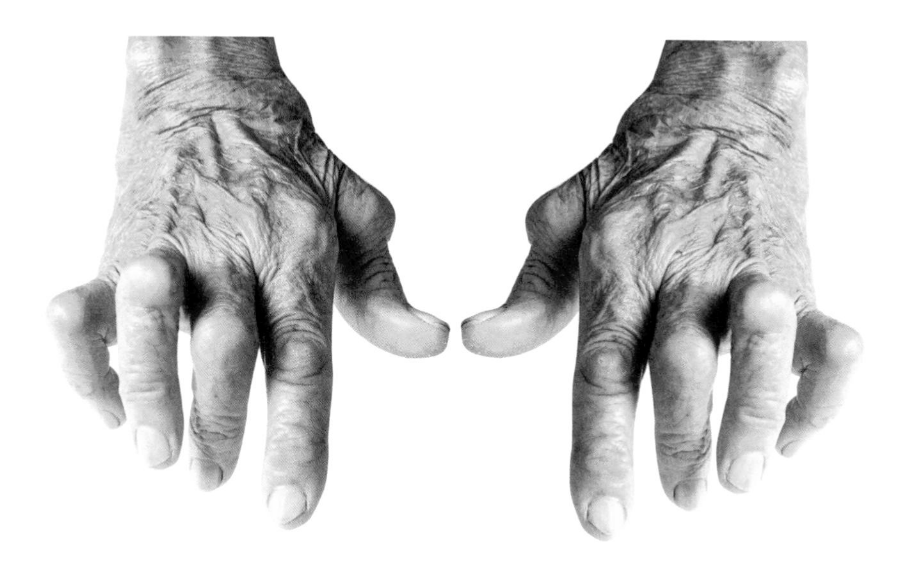

C) Trigger Finger

Trigger finger is a condition characterized by the finger (and sometimes the thumb) being stuck in a flexed position. This can be painful and functionally problematic.

The cause is usually associated with repeated use and the resulting inflammation of the tendons. Tendons naturally flow through an outside covering called a sheath. This is sort of like a string gliding through a drinking straw. When the straw gets narrowed or the string enlarges,

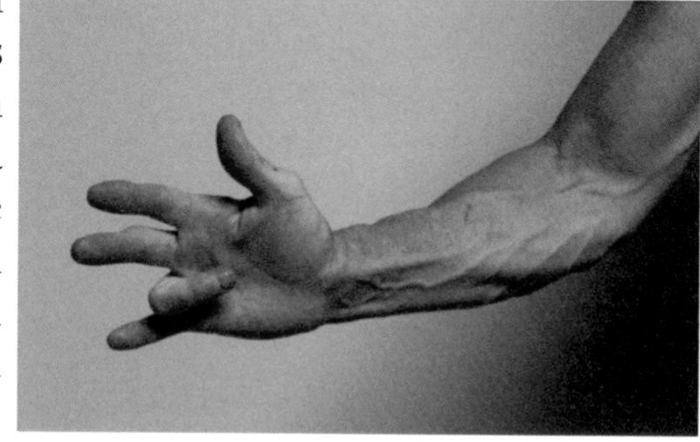

the motion is disturbed. There are no X-ray or lab tests for this one. Clinical diagnosis is simple based on patient presentation.

Treatment includes rest and sometimes splinting of the affected finger. Ice, NSAIDs and natural anti-inflammatories like turmeric and ginger can help. Severe cases can be treated with steroid shots, but make sure this is performed by an orthopedist to avoid tendon damage. Surgery to free up the entrapped tendon is very simple with great results.

CHAPTER TEN

Health Care and Alternative Treatments

My Thought Process

As we age, visits to the doctor become all too common. All of us consider alternative treatments for what's ailing us, but how many of these treatments are helpful and how many are not what they are cracked up to be? In this chapter, I will give you my opinion, based on 30 years of chiropractic practice. My insight is forged by a strong sense of logic and a complete inability to just "believe in" anything. If someone says this works a certain way, I need to know why. I'm not a big fan of others' theories or philosophies, not to mention that the science community is so corrupt with politics and agenda-driven studies that I am initially skeptical of their conclusions.

I will express my thoughts on everything from acupuncture to yoga. This is largely opinion, based on my own philosophy. I have found two basic principles of life that formulate the majority of my thought processes.

First, follow the money. When something really works, consumers will beat down the door to get it. If something is continually vilified in the media and yet still prospers, there has to be something to it. On the other hand, when something is promoted endlessly in the news with the same old fear tactics, I wonder if money is the driver. Think about the annual news report we get that states how bad the upcoming flu season is going to be and vehemently encourages us to get our shots. It always puzzles me how pharmaceutical companies can predict an upcoming bad flu season. That is about as easy as predicting the weather next year.

The next principle of reasoning I use is controversial, so please prepare yourself. I believe in God, or a creator, or a higher being, however you'd like to phrase it. Yes, I know that sounds crazy for some of you. With that in mind, when I come across news that proclaims potential miracle cures from improbable places, I always think to myself "Would God do that?" For example, would God put the secret to joint health on the belly of a killer shark? Would God put the secret to curing cancer in the seed of a berry located on an island 500 miles south of Indonesia? Probably not. Shark cartilage doesn't do anything to help regenerate joints, and I can't even remember the name of the expensive, obscure berry that was supposed to cure cancer.

I will refer to the placebo effect several times in this chapter. A placebo is anything given to a patient that is represented to be a real drug when, in fact, it's not a drug at all. This fake drug is given to a group of people while the real drug is administered to another. Neither group knows who has the real drug and who received the placebo. The response of the placebo group is then measured against the group that took the real medication. Some in the placebo group will experience a benefit while others will experience negative effects. These effects are called the placebo effect. This test shows the role of the human mind in making someone sick or better. Let's take a look at some alternative treatments and see which ones are the real deal.

Acupunture

I'm going to be up front from the get-go on this one. I'm not a fan. I still haven't had one acupuncturist explain to me how poking holes in the skin at specific points medically accomplishes anything. I think this treatment is a classic example of the placebo effect. I have heard rumors that eastern "medicine practitioners" perform open heart surgery without general anesthesia. Instead, they stick a few needles in their patient's skin and – mysteriously – the patient doesn't feel their chest being split apart. This just does not happen. Once again, follow the money. If you try hard enough, you can find an acupuncturist, but you don't see them on every block like you do chiropractors or physical therapists. And there's a reason for that. It doesn't work. The placebo effect only goes so far.

CBD Oil

CBD oil is the newest rage in the holistic medicine community since the legalization of medical marijuana. The oil is derived from the flowers and buds of the hemp plants. However, CBD oil doesn't contain THC, the intoxicating component of the marijuana plant. Proponents claim the oil can help with anything from anxiety to sleeplessness. Studies have shown CBD oil to have some positive effects on many conditions including managing epilepsy. The oil clearly has some chemical effect on our body because it can interact with pharmaceutical drugs, particularly anti-epileptic medicine. CBD oil can increase the effects of sedative medications. CBD can slow down how the body metabolizes certain drugs making the drugs stay in our system for a longer time. This can be useful with certain drugs and present problems with other medications such as blood thinners. Therefore, if you take prescription medication consult your medical doctor to see if it's safe to take CBD. Over time, we might find this oil to be of use as an accelerant to certain medications enhancing their effectiveness.

One thing I find troubling about CBD oil is the quality control in the manufacturing process. Less than half of all the CBD oil products actually contain the amount of CBD stated on the bottle. Another problem could be toxicity to the liver. The oil does raise liver enzymes, indicating a potentially mild toxic effect on the body. The other problem I have with accepting CBD oil's validation as a medical treatment is that none of the favorable studies contain a control group. Could this be another example of the placebo effect? I'm not convinced either way on this one yet. I have had a lot of credible patients relate positive experiences with CBD. I'm cautiously optimistic with this one.

Chiropractic

Chiropractic is a branch of the healing arts. Its basic premise is that the spine houses the nervous system. At every level of the spine, peripheral nerves exit to their respective tissues. These nerves control all functions of the body – everything from muscle tissue to organ functions. Mechanical dysfunction at any level could affect the ability of the nerve to do its duty. Structural misalignment could result in communication problems between the brain and the body. Poor spinal alignment could cause pressure that diminishes a nerve's impulses to its designated destination. This issue can also negatively affect the nervous system's ability to relay a message from its origin in the body to the brain. If nerve transmission is altered, things might not work as well as they should. It's not that complicated – any structural misalignment presents a subtle form of stress to the body. I could never figure out why this simple idea was so hard to grasp in the medical community. Some doctors think nerves work perfectly or not at all, when in fact it isn't necessarily black or white. There could be shades of gray. At one time or another, every one of us has fallen asleep on their arm, only to awaken with it being numb and momentarily disabled. Also, who hasn't had numbness or tingling in their legs because they were crossed for too long? What happens when you get off the compressed arm or leg? The nerve starts to work again and function is restored. It's as simple as that. Additionally, we have to consider that there are nerves that control blood pressure, balance, digestion, and organ functions. Any of these structures can have similar issues if compromised. The healing possibilities of nerve decompression are endless.

Don't get me wrong. Nerve compression is not the sole cause of all disease. However, it is reasonable to consider it as one of several factors. Genetics also play a role in disease, as do environmental influences and exposure. The importance of diet and nutrition in fighting disease – or even causing it – can't be overstated. The real truth of the matter is that we are finding out that it's a combination of all of the above – a combination of A, B and C. For example, if the exposure was the sole cause of a disease, why doesn't everyone that smokes get lung cancer? Conversely, why do some people that don't smoke get lung cancer? If you have a genetic predisposition for getting lung cancer, it is even worse for you to smoke than it is for everyone else. Another example: if genetics are the sole cause of disease, why wouldn't identical twins with identical genes both die from the same natural cause? I've seen many patients that were identical twins suffer from completely different disorders. Lastly, if nutrition was the sole cause of disease, why do I see farmers regularly in my office that are 90 years old who eat bacon, eggs, and scrapple, yet don't suffer from coronary artery disease? I could go on and on, but you get the point. To complicate matters more, we are finding that disease is not only a combination of factors; it can also be dependent on the order of exposure to each factor.

As mentioned earlier in this book, the single greatest thing that a chiropractor does is restore motion. As we age, tissues degenerate and subsequently harden. This phenomenon manifests itself in the form of loss of motion and fixation. Inducing motion into these fixed areas helps restore function. Chiropractors are trained in short-lever techniques that minimize collateral tissue involvement. Specificity is the key to motion restoration without injury.

Another focus of chiropractic care is the maintenance of platform structure and making sure the leg lengths and the pelvis are level. Chiropractic care focuses on mechanical restoration through manual movements of the body's parts. These adjustments to the frame accomplish better mechanics during motion. Better motion and optimal body positioning result in a decreased likelihood of injury. This makes complete sense. Yet, the Wikipedia definition of chiropractic at the time of this book's writing is rife with negative innuendo, such as "claims that are not scientifically based," "its foundation is at odds with mainstream medicine," and, of course, the obligatory "chiropractors are not medical doctors." I've been asked to testify as an expert witness in several personal injury and workman's compensation cases. The lawyer representing the other side always asks me the rubber stamp question, "You are not a medical doctor, is that correct?" Despite the attorneys' attempts to diminish chiropractic's legitimacy with negative connotations, I've won every case because the results spoke for themselves.

Follow the money. Chiropractic malpractice insurance cost is 1/50th of an orthopedic surgeon and 1/10th of a general practitioner. So, who here is dangerous? Insurance companies play no favorites.

Getting routine chiropractic maintenance care ensures better health. I get adjusted every month and have found that to be a perfect schedule for me. Everyone is different; depending on age and physical condition, treatment frequency is variable. Over time, your needs can be determined with the help of your chiropractor.

Homeopathy

This practice started in the late-1700s. Homeopathy is rooted in the theory that "like cures like." It was based on the thought that things which produce the symptoms of a disease in healthy people can cure sufferers of the actual ailment. For example: if you have an allergy that makes your eyes water, take onion since onions can make your eyes water when freshly cut. Needless to say, this has been proven not to work. Even worse, homeopathic treatments can cause ailments. As interesting as it is to look at old homeopathic medicine bottles to see what was in them, you can understand why people lived only until 40 in those times. You will need a healthy dose of the placebo effect to honestly believe these remedies will work.

Follow the money. I don't even know where to find a homeopathic practitioner.

Hypnosis Therapy

Now we have a tricky one. Hypnotherapy uses concentration and heightened focus of attention to achieve a state of consciousness where the person blocks out their surroundings. With the help of a trained therapist, suggestions can help someone recall painful thoughts that have been blocked or memories that have been hidden by the conscious mind. After seeing people get hypnotized, my initial skepticism that anyone could be hypnotized was gone. There are two types of hypnotic therapy: analysis therapy and suggestion therapy.

Analysis therapy focuses on putting the patient in a hypnotic state to explore repressed memories. The psychology behind this is to find if there is a mental reason for the patient's illness or pain. The jury is still out on whether or not the pain is in the patient's head. Psychosomatic events are noted clinically and are hard to ignore from a physician's point of view. If the cause of the patient's pain has psychiatric roots, it's reasonable to suggest that hypnotherapy treatment could help.

Suggestion therapy might have less value. Once under hypnosis, the patient is given suggestions to help a particular bad habit, like smoking. Others have said that it can aid in the perception of pain. The use of suggestions under hypnosis to enhance the capacity for feeling less discomfort is unconfirmed.

One of the commonly agreed-upon drawbacks to hypnotherapy is that the treatment can aid in the formation of false memories. If the therapist uses leading or suggestive questions, the patient can recall things that in reality didn't happen.

All of this is to say, "Show me the results." I have found very few people that responded to smoking cessation therapy via hypnotherapy. I can't recall anyone telling me they received any mental health benefit or decreased pain benefit from hypnotherapy. So, if it barks like a dog and has a tail like a dog, it's probably a dog. I think this one is a dog.

Massage Therapy

We don't need to spend a lot of time on this one. I see little downside to getting a massage. It's useful for stress relief, relaxation of muscle tissue, and increased flexibility which can yield better all around performance. However, there is no reason to be brutalized when getting a massage. If you are black and blue the next day, your masseuse is going too heavy.

The only real concern with massage therapy is if there are underlying vascular issues. Varicose veins should be left alone. Massage therapists are trained to recognize these situations.

When choosing a massage therapist I recommend finding one with a diploma in Medical Massage with licensure from the state. With little downside and a lot of upside, I give massage therapy two thumbs up.

Magnetic Therapy

There's not much to say about this one. The theory behind this one is that strategically positioned magnets on a person can influence the meridians or magnetic fields which allegedly control their body. The problem is that the magnets aren't strong enough to do anything. Not to mention, we are surrounded by magnetic fields all day. In this regard, the body is not a mystery. Our physiology is easy to effect. All we have to do is put an ice cube on your forearm, let it sit there for 5 minutes. Once removed, you can see a nice, red mark right where the ice was. You can clearly see that the ice caused an effect on the body's chemistry. Magnets placed on our skin cause no skin color changes one way or another. There is no measurable evidence of any effect on muscles or nerves, either. Not to mention, the cost associated with some of these items is prohibitive. The placebo effect is your only chance for magnets to help. Don't waste your money.

Medical Marijuana

Pot has been around since the third millennium B.C.! It's been popular and vilified through the ages – who can forget the 1936 propaganda movie Reefer Madness? In the interest of full disclosure, I'm going to be upfront and say that I wasn't inhaling pot about the same time Bill Clinton didn't inhale... Well, at least since the late '70s! My college chemical experimentation was limited to late night parties and the resultant effect of a phone call to have a pizza delivered.

The positive effects of marijuana include appetite stimulation, decreased blood pressure, pain relief, decreased anxiety, enhanced sensory perceptions, and decreased nausea with cancer treatments. The negative effects of smoking weed may include a somewhat altered sense, reduced ambition, paranoia, increased heart rate, and panic attacks.

I might part from a lot of my conservative ideologies on this one. I think this gets one thumbs up. If it's recreational use you are looking for, you are dealing with the same upsides and downsides as alcohol. But from a medicinal point of view, I see way more benefits than detractors. Effect on pain management has been proven. The decrease in blood pressure clearly helps with conditions like glaucoma. Increased appetite can be useful in maintaining proper nutrition and health when dealing with a multitude of disorders. Maybe this one has stayed around so long for the recreational benefits, but I think it's worth a try when suffering any chronic pain disorder.

PRP and Stem Cell Treatment

PRP stands for "platelet rich plasma." Platelets are the component of blood that helps with blood clotting. Additionally, these cells are loaded with proteins and growth factors that help regenerate tissue. The procedure entails drawing blood and putting it into a centrifuge. Since the platelets are heavier than the other blood cells, the platelets will aggregate at the bottom of the test tube. They will then be drawn from there and injected into diseased or injured tissue. This procedure is relatively new but the results have been dramatic.

Follow the money. Just 5 years ago, there were a handful of doctors in the entire country doing this procedure. Now, every city has doctors performing this procedure. I like the logic behind this one, and more importantly, I have seen the positive clinical results. I think PRP and other forms of stem cell therapy are the future of orthopedic medicine. The only downside is that PRP is a little expensive. Stem cell treatment is very expensive. Both of these work and are worth a try.

Taping

Kinesiology taping is different from athletic taping. Athletic taping is used to stabilize an injured area. This tape is removed as soon as the athletic activity is completed. Kinesiology taping is used for a decrease in pain, possible dispersal of swelling, and an increase in circulation, and can also be kept on the body for one to four days. The Kinesiology tape is elastic and meant to be stretched when placing over a muscle.

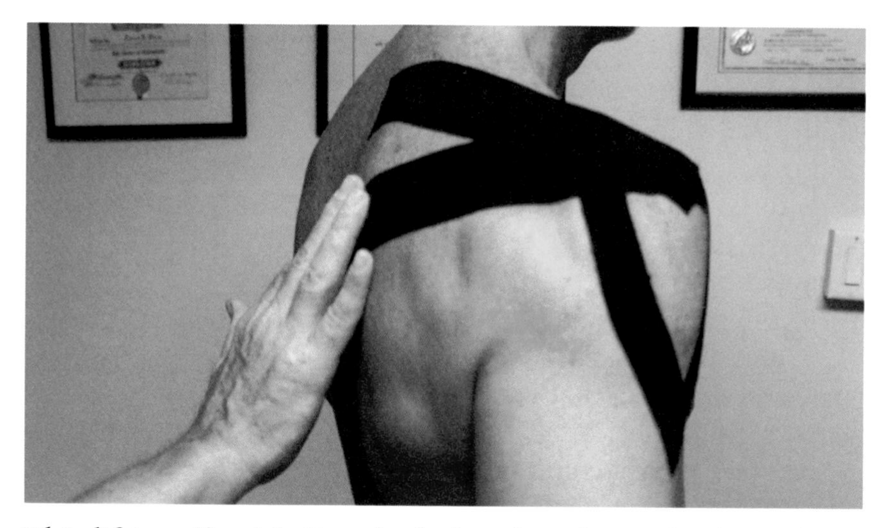

This lifting effect is believed to help reduce discomfort by enabling more venous drainage. The same vacuum-like effect might help release byproducts of physical exercise, such as lactic acid, thereby providing more endurance, enhanced performance, and possibly quicker recovery. The results speak for themselves. Most using the kinesiology tape have found it helps. I think there's little-to-no doubt about the pain reduction component. Whether or not there's agreement with the mechanism of action doesn't matter. It clearly works and I suggest you give it a try. I put some videos up on **DrDeanWolf.com** to show how to tape commonly injured structures.

Vaccinations

There's probably no topic that will create more controversy than this one. Let's throw out emotion and just discuss some basic facts. The basic thought behind vaccinations is to give the patient a super small amount of a bug, against which the body's immune system then develops an antibody. I think there is validity to the mechanisms of this argument. However, there are two things that trouble me greatly about vaccinations: the gross inappropriate use of them and the complete failure to scientifically test them via the most basic of all scientific tenets, the double blind study.

Let's discuss the inappropriate use first. We will stick to just one example because an entire book could be written on this topic alone. We will use the tetanus vaccine as an example since it's a popular vaccination. Clostridium Tetani is a bacteria that is cultured in the large intestine from a horse and some other animals. Tetanus is a very wimpy bacteria. It only survives in a damp, moist anaerobic environment. Air kills it. Hence, the rusty nail – to get tetanus, it has to be introduced into your body anaerobically, through a puncture wound. So, if you were to step on a rusty nail that was covered in horse manure, you could get a tetanus infection. It wasn't much more than a century ago that horses were a common vehicle of transportation. It wasn't unimaginable to step on a nail that was covered in horse manure. In today's fast-paced world, the risk of exposure, combined with all the right conditions needed, makes it unlikely to even have the slightest risk of infection. A few years ago, I had a crush injury to my foot. A big piece of steel in a commercial cooler fell on my foot, resulting in several fractures and a first-class ticket to the emergency room. The very first thing the ER doctor attempted was to give me a tetanus shot. When I refused it, he looked at me like I had two heads. When I explained my position, I realized he didn't know the basic etiology of the tetanus infection. I gave him the same disturbed look.

We are so brainwashed with fear mongering through the media by the pharmaceutical industry. It's thought of as sophistry if you question putting a toxin in your body. Simple logic can prove the herd immunity effect to be false. To prove my point, think of this: there is one subset of our population that will not get their tetanus booster shots. That's right, adult men. Men don't listen to their bodies and don't go to doctors. No matter how hard the media tries to convince men to go to the doctor to get their shots, they just will not. So, the promoters of these vaccinations are stuck inducing fear into the parts of the population that will respond with the least resistance: senior citizens and children. If these vaccinations are so critically important to herd immunity, then where is the outbreak of tetanus, whooping cough and diphtheria in adult males? Something to think about.

Lastly, the double blind study is the most fundamental principle of all science. Nevertheless, no double blind studies are performed when it comes to vaccination research. The arguments against doing double blind studies on vaccinations lack any logic.

I had a patient that wanted to have his daughter looked at by a pediatrician, but was having trouble finding one because she wasn't vaccinated. Another one of my patients was a pediatrician, and so I proceeded to give him a call. I asked him if he would see her as a patient. He told me that their office policy was to see only vaccinated patients with no exceptions. I told him I respected his decision. He wanted to explain his position, but I told him that it wasn't necessary. He insisted and explained that if he chose to see unvaccinated patients, it could pose a risk to his other patients – you know, the vaccinated ones! This reasoning completely escaped me. Not only does this argument make no sense, it brings into question the effectiveness of the vaccine itself.

Everyone has to follow their own sense of judgment on this one. I think you can make a reasonable argument for the shingles vaccination if you're over 60 and had chickenpox, or if you are traveling to a country where exposure becomes an issue. On the other hand, I completely disagree with getting the flu shot. When the Obama administration decided to declare a national emergency because two people were infected with swine flu, it took the pharmaceutical machine months to come up with a vaccination and then longer to put into place a pipeline to manufacture and distribute the vaccine. Keep in mind, it took that long even when the science community knew what flu vaccine to work on. What bothers me the most about the flu vaccine is that there is no way we can determine what strain of flu will be prevalent next year. Not to mention, such a large percentage of the patients I see get sick after the vaccination. Our immune system has only so many bullets. I don't see any reason to use any of our immunity weapons on the flu.

Yoga

I like yoga and any other form of activity programs that produce increased range of motion, stretching, and exercising. There are obvious physical and mental benefits when participating in Zumba, Pilates, and spinning classes, just to name a few. The fountain of youth is flexibility and activity. If you don't use it, you lose it.

Conclusion

The secret to being in great shape is a combination of everything in this book. We have to eat strategically in conjunction with training both aerobically and with weights. In addition, specific supplementation should be taken to fit your body's needs. The use of tools, like orthotics or heel lifts, to help our bodies maintain good mechanics can't be overstated. Treat injuries by way of multi-tiered approaches that can include bracing, chiropractic care, ice, eccentric exercise activity and nutritional support.

People are shaped, molded, motivated, and inspired through personal experiences and teachings. Every individual is unique and precious. So, while I laid out information for your consideration, you will have to determine the right prescriptive regimen for yourself. I wholeheartedly believe with patience, determination, and the applications found in this book, your transformation has just begun.

A diamond is a piece of coal that finished the job...